True Birth

A Compilation of Real Birth Stories

First edition

MARIKA JEZIOREK

www.FeelGoodGivingBirth.com

Printed in the United States of America.

First edition.

Proofreading by Weronika King.

Cover picture submitted by Mary Beth Trendos.

Names, characters, places and incidents are either the product of the author's imagination or are used fictitiously, and any resemblance to any actual persons, living or dead, events, or locales is entirely coincidental.

The Content is not intended to be a substitute for professional medical advice, diagnosis, or treatment, nor is the material to be considered an offer, a solicitation for an offer to sell or buy, or an endorsement, a recommendation or a sponsorship of any company, product or service. Always seek medical advice for any questions regarding your pregnancy, labor, and delivery. If you think you may have a medical emergency, call your doctor or emergency services immediately.

Published by Advancing Thought.

ISBN: 978-0-9938356-0-5

For my family and friends – thank you for your love, support, and encouragement.

To all those working towards making childbirth a peaceful, joyful, and empowering experience, where women feel safe and secure, and where their rights are respected, thank you from the bottom of my heart.

Contents

Introduction

As the title of the book suggests, this book will explore true birth. It will outline the multifaceted dimensions of childbirth by examining both the personal experience of the mother, as well as the evidence-based research surrounding various childbirth issues. While stripping away the layers of culture and one's deeply-founded understanding of birth may not be possible, this book will attempt to show 'birth' as it is, by examining it as it is known and as it is experienced by the main actors – mothers.

You will read about how mothers approached childbirth, what they did to prepare, and how they managed unexpected circumstances. You will read about their reflection, and you will be privy to short interviews with the mothers where they explain what they liked most and least about their birth, and what they feel a mother should know or do before she gives birth.

There are hospital births, home births, and births somewhere in between. There are vaginal births, and C-section births. There are joyful births, and there are sad births. There are empowering births where the mothers felt strong, in control, and fearless, and there are violent births where women felt disrespected, violated, and ignored. Where they were ridiculed for wanting a natural birth, and criticized for being 'selfish' for wanting to try alternative methods. There are births where women's rights in childbirth were protected and enforced, and there are births where rights of the mother were nonexistent and irrelevant.

Their stories may differ, and they may all be unique, but as you will see, all mothers featured in this book have something in common. They all have hope. They all possess and highlight positivity. They all stand in solidarity with the mother next to them, and encourage her to be fearless. To be strong. They encourage women to take back their rights, to demand that they be respected, and that they, as women in childbirth, be supported and listened to.

These mothers stress the crucial aspect of being educated and ready. Expectant mothers need to understand how their body works during childbirth. What is and what is not normal. What is recommended based on nature and physiology, and what is recommended based on the convenience of the health care provider. Women need to understand that where they give birth, and with whose help they give birth (if any), will influence their birth. They need to choose wisely.

> *Women need to understand that where they give birth, and with whose help they give birth, will influence their birth. They need to choose wisely.*

By preparing the body, mind, and soul, and by choosing the environment and health care providers that will work best for them, women will play a significant role in their childbirth. When fear is present, or when you are insufficiently prepared, you will not have the desire or tools that are necessary to push for the birth that you want.

Please enjoy this book for all the heart-warming stories that it contains, and the insightful articles provided by our wonderful contributors. If you are an expectant mom, we hope you are well-reminded that you are strong and incredible, and that you have the right to influence your childbirth. If you are an expectant father, we hope you learn about the importance of this event for the mother, and how you can provide the support she needs to push for what she wants. If you already had a wonderful birth, we hope you are reminded about the positivity and happiness that you experienced. If you had a sad birth, or a birth that you are having trouble discussing, we hope these mothers provide the advice or supporting words that you may need to find closure. If you are a grandparent, sibling, or friend, we hope you better understand childbirth, and the importance of discussing this event. We hope all of you further the discourse of childbirth, and never ignore it as an irrelevant milestone that is best left unspoken of. We hope you rejoice in the birth of a baby, and of a mother, while recognizing that the way a mother experiences birth, and remembers it, is important.

Childbirth discourse is upon us, but it is up to every one of us to guide the discourse into a positive interpretation, which showcases the sheer power of women, and presents them as strong individuals who have the right to birth in a respectful and supportive environment.

Pure Bliss

Before we divide up the birth stories by location, let us examine births that were simply pure bliss. There births, which were empowering to the mothers, were full of joy, and were truly spectacular. It is possible to enjoy birth. It is possible to be full of love and joy during childbirth. It is possible to have the birth that you envision, whether in a hospital, or at home. This can be your reality, and it is attainable.

■■

Karin Ritter

Karin's story shows us that it is absolutely possible to feel good giving birth. There is raw power and strength. There is no fear or panic. There is complete calm and tranquility. Karin prepared for her childbirth by practicing hot yoga and by learning as much as possible in advance about the physical and mental components of giving birth. She underwent hypnosis, and had the birth she envisioned for herself. With knowledge and understanding, the expectant mother is well-prepared to embark on this remarkable journey into motherhood.

HYPNO-WHAT?!

"Every emotion, every feeling, every step of the process was amazing to me."

My son was born exactly on his due date at 1:36 pm. I had prepared for a Hypnobabies birth for the two months leading up to his birthday. My friends laughed at me, "Hypno-what?!" One insisted, "You will WANT the epidural. Trust me!" I knew myself better than anyone and I knew that what I wanted was to have him naturally, without any medical intervention.

Towards the end of my pregnancy, I told my mother that I was pretty sure that when I went into labor, it would be around four in the morning, because that was when he was always most active. He would wake me up like clockwork every day at that time. On Thursday, I went for my weekly appointment, and my doctor told me I was about 2-3 cm dilated. The following Saturday, I spent about two hours walking slowly up and down the stairs at my own turtle pace trying to get things moving. Later that day, I was bleeding a little and then the following morning, my son let me know that he was on his way.

I woke up a few times with pressure waves (contractions), but in my sleepy haze, I didn't comprehend that I was in labor, so I kept trying to go back to sleep. When I finally realized what my body was telling me, I went downstairs and washed the dishes. Then, I went to my computer to finish up some changes in my birth plan. I was a bit hungry, so I ate some yogurt and toast, but I immediately had to run to the bathroom and proceeded to vomit. This actually woke up my husband, who came downstairs and asked if I was all right. Between heaves, I told him that the baby would be making his entrance into the world that day!

I went upstairs to take a warm shower to try and relax. While I was in there, I asked my husband to call my doctor to tell him I was in labor. Since it was Sunday, it went to the voicemail, and the doctor on call gave us a call back. When I got out of the shower, I turned on my Hypnobabies birthing tracks on my phone and put my earphones in (they stayed in my ears until my son was born). It was around 9 am when the doctor called, and at that point, I had been having my contractions for a little over four hours. I had been clocking my birthing waves on an app on my phone to track my progress. My contractions were lasting about 45 seconds every three minutes. After I relayed this information to the doctor, she told me to wait another hour because she liked her "first-time-mommy" patients to be at least 4 cm dilated before arriving at the hospital. I hung up the phone and remembered that my doctor had told me I was about 2-3 cm three days prior, so I made the decision to head to the hospital, as I was sure I was at least 4 cm and exactly as the doctor preferred.

Every time a birthing wave approached, I just stared out the window using my Hypnobabies techniques and kept my breathing regular.

Arriving at the hospital around 10 am, we went to triage where they checked my progress. They were surprised to see that I was already at 7 cm, even though this was my first baby. They admitted me right away and my husband requested IV fluids for me, as he thought I would be dehydrated from being previously ill. We went to my Labor & Delivery Room, which had a beautiful view of the Pacific Ocean. Every time a birthing wave approached, I just stared out the window using my Hypnobabies techniques and kept my breathing regular. We had forgotten my birth plan in the car, but my nurse Josette, who had experience with Hypnobabies, was absolutely amazing, and assured me I would know when it would be time to push.

My water had not broken yet, but I suddenly understood what Josette was talking about, as this new feeling was much different than the pressure waves I had been experiencing all morning. She checked, and said that I was 10 cm dilated, and that I could start pushing. She called the doctor to give her an update. I requested to have the head of the bed raised and got on my knees and leaned over the back of the bed. I started pushing a little after noon. I was slightly disappointed when my water broke, because I thought it would be neat if my baby was born in the caul. When the doctor arrived, she could tell I was getting a little tired, so she told me it would be easier for me to lay on my back and push. My husband told me he could see the baby's head. I was getting a little tired, so I took a few moments to rest. Josette said that since it had been a while since my last contraction, the next one would be the "big push."

After two more pushes, his head came out. His shoulders were stuck, so the doctor maneuvered to release them. She asked me if I wanted to pull him out on my own. I was so excited! I reached down, grabbed my baby, and pulled him up to my chest. My husband told me that I kept repeating "Hi Baby!" over and over again. I immediately fell in love with all 9 pounds, 15 ounces of him. Afterwards, Josette asked me if I was an athlete because my heart rate stayed so low and regular in between contractions. I told her that it was probably because I

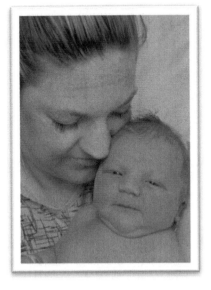

had practiced hot yoga up until the eighth month of my pregnancy.

What did you like most and least about your childbirth experience?

There was nothing about my birthing experience that I didn't love. Every emotion, every feeling, every step of the process was amazing to me. I spent a lot of time learning about the birthing process and about what happens to the body during birth.

There was nothing about my birthing experience that I didn't love.

What would you tell an expectant mother to better prepare her for childbirth?

I think all women should spend a few months learning about the chemical and physical changes that are going on in their bodies during pregnancy, during birth, and thereafter. It was really beneficial for me to have this awareness, along with my yoga practice and the Hypnobabies technique – I felt really prepared for childbirth.

■■■

Tamika Newman

Tamika had exactly the birth she wanted. She felt happy and empowered. She felt secure and comfortable. She loved it all. She understood the need to trust her own body, and she encourages all expectant parents to choose their caregiver wisely, as this decision will most certainly influence their experience. Her story is beautiful and shows women that they have the ability to influence the way they give birth. Tamika's birth was simply normal, yet absolutely magical.

The Birth of Imogen Rose

"My birth was simply amazing... I felt so empowered."

On Friday, March 14th, 2014, at 41w 5d pregnant, I woke up and was an emotional mess! I had my midwife appointment at 11 am and had asked my hubby Ben to come, as I needed his extra love and support. I was quite stressed at what would happen once I hit that 42 weeks' mark, and the rigmarole that I would have to deal with once I went "overdue." My midwife offered a membrane sweep, and I agreed.

About 30 minutes after my sweep, I got my first contraction. Driving home I got another one, and another once we got home. I started thinking it was just a reaction to having the sweep, and didn't think too much of it. I cuddled Isla to sleep for her nap. While standing up, I had another contraction. By the time Ben got home, which was around 2:15 pm, I had had a few contractions that definitely felt a little more "real" this time. We decided to call my mum and ask her to collect Isla.

At 3 pm, the contractions were coming every 3 minutes on the dot, and lasted between 45 and 60 seconds. I was having to vocalize through them. At this point, I really didn't believe I was in labor, as I had experienced so many false starts. However, these were regular contractions, and I was having to stop, breathe, and vocalize.

My midwife arrived with all her equipment around 3:45 pm. I think I even asked her whether she thought it was real. She gave me a funny look and smiled. At about 4:10 pm, the second midwife arrived. It's quite funny to think about it now, but at the time, I was still in disbelief. I couldn't believe this was really happening.

We had closed all the curtains to make the house as dark as possible. Three of our neighbours decided it was the perfect time to mow their lawns; we were serenaded with the sound of mowers - cutting the grass in unison!

The midwives took up residence on the couch, had a cup of tea, while playing some games on their iPad, and let me labor away! I felt so calm and super relaxed. I was laughing and chatting between my contractions. My midwife would listen in to bubs every now and then, and she was doing absolutely well! Her heart rate did not drop once. I had years of experience, listening to fetal heart rates and caring for women, so I knew she was perfectly happy. I was also getting kicks and jabs in the ribs both during, and between, contractions. My midwife would come over every now and then and rub some essential oils (clary sage) onto my back, and

I was still laughing and joking in between contractions.

remind me to relax my shoulders. Although her presence was felt, I was calm, in control, and didn't need anyone at that point.

While it felt lovely to relax and float in the pool, it didn't give me as much relief as I was expecting. Looking back, I now know this was because I was hitting transition and probably around 7-8 cm dilated. I guess nowhere is really comfortable, but I was still laughing and joking in between contractions. The midwives thought it was hilarious that I was so happy even though I wasn't far off from having a baby!

I only stopped laughing/joking about 15-20 minutes before Imogen was born. At this point, I got into my little zone, and gave my hubby's hands a good squeeze during contractions. I was super vocal, as I drew down my inner cavewoman.

I remember feeling like it would be a good idea to give a little push with a contraction, but I didn't have an overwhelming urge to push just yet. I started to push with contractions, but it was different than the normal 'purple pushing' scenario that happens in a hospital. It was a bit of noise (push) for every minute and move. I remember getting a cramp in my legs, and having to change position. I was moving around the pool quite a bit, similar to a lion pacing in a cage.

I felt like I pushed forever, but my midwife assures me it was at most 10 minutes from the first push to our baby being born. I remember giving a push and feeling this pop/gush of fluid, and sure enough my waters had broken. It was the weirdest feeling as it happened in the water. I had a little smile to myself, as obviously my baby was nowhere near overdue and she was just right!

I stood up briefly until the next contraction hit, but then I got back in that water, as it was obviously what I needed to get bubs into the right position. For the next contraction, I got up on all fours, over the side of the pool, and felt bubs' head literally drop into my pelvis. It was a sensation like no other, as I knew I was so close to having my baby, but the feeling of this super hard ball stretching inside me was something else.

I don't feel I can put into words how truly powerful birth can be. I felt so empowered.

During the next contraction, I felt a lot of stinging and stretching. I put my hand down, and felt a decent amount of super soft hair. With the next contraction, I birthed her head. The midwife suggested I "give another little push to birth her chin." I did as instructed, and thought that was a little unusual at the time, but then I saw the size of her cheeks and understood why! Between the birth of her head and the next contraction, my midwife told me to just open my legs a little wider. I then felt her shoulders turn – boy, did I feel that! I then slowly birthed her shoulders, which came out beautifully, followed slowly by her body.

I turned and scooped her up out of the water, and felt nothing but sheer elation and joy. I had done everything I had set out to achieve. I had my beautiful home water birth! Our gorgeous Imogen Rose was born at 7:13 pm. I scooped her into my arms and she was so super peaceful - it was like she didn't even know she had been born. She was pink, had a great heart rate and tone, but wasn't breathing or crying yet. I was totally calm as I knew she was still attached to her placenta/cord, which was providing all the oxygen she needed. After about 2 minutes she let out a tiny little cry and then started to open her eyes. At one point, I remember thinking about her sex. I looked and saw she was a girl. It was a strange feeling, as we didn't officially *know* her sex beforehand, but I somehow knew that she was a little girl all along.

Within 10 minutes of her birth, my little champion hopped onto the breast and had her first feed. The midwives and Ben helped me out of the pool, and as I stood up, my placenta literally fell out! A lovely big juicy healthy placenta with absolutely no sign of 'post maturity' whatsoever. I hopped on the couch, where I snuggled and fed my gorgeous little cherub. The midwives had a look to see if there was any damage, and I was elated to hear that I didn't have any tearing!

After around an hour and a half of skin-to-skin, several feedings and snuggles, I decided it was time to weigh Imogen and cut her cord. Can you imagine the surprise for everyone when she weighed in at 4,620 g, 58 cm long, and had a head circumference of 36.5 cm! Not long after Imogen was weighed, my gorgeous big girl arrived to meet her little sister for the very first time. She was so excited to have a sister. She came over and we all snuggled on the couch, while Imogen had another feed.

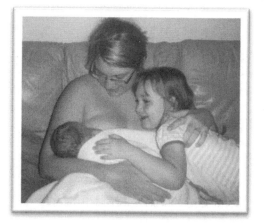

What did you like most about your childbirth experience?

My birth was simply amazing. I don't feel I can put into words how truly powerful birth can be. I felt so empowered. I loved the fact that I labored and birthed totally unhindered and undisturbed. My midwife did not touch my daughter until two hours after birth. I also felt so safe and secure by being in my own home, having people who believed in birth and whom I thoroughly trusted, watching over me.

I also felt so safe and secure by being in my own home, having people who believed in birth and whom I thoroughly trusted, watching over me.

What did you like least about your childbirth experience?

Nothing. I would do it all over again a thousand times.

What would you tell an expectant mother to better prepare her for childbirth?

The birth of your child will stick with you forever and will influence your parenting journey. You need to prepare before conception! Learn to love and trust your body and the birth process. You also need to be very cautious in choosing your caregiver. Choose someone who believes in birth and who doesn't see it as a 'medical condition' that needs to be fixed. Interview many and choose one who feels right for you.

Your Most Important Labor Support

Sarah Clark

My first birth was a 50+ hour event that ended in a midwife-assisted natural hospital birth. I was struck by two things. First, I felt simply lucky. I had a great midwife assigned to me, a quiet but kind nurse, a childbirth educator who walked me through the process, and a husband who was perfect. Second, I was overwhelmed with a feeling of my own awesomeness. I had never done anything in my life that was that hard, that long, that taxing or that empowering. I truly felt that I could do anything.

That sense of awe in my own ability stuck with me and carried me through many days of motherhood and many new challenges that came through the years after. Birth didn't just happen to me, I triumphed over it. There is nothing that compares to what it did for my feelings of worth and confidence. There were no other options after – I would somehow help other women have this same life-changing experience.

We live in a world where you can hire somebody for just about anything. This is as true with birth as anything else. There are doctors, midwives, doulas, childbirth educators, nurses, chiropractors, placenta encapsulation specialists and the list goes on; all people you can bring into your circle of birth to help support you. You can even take a birth class to help your partner be prepared and wonderful at your birth (this is my specialty and I love it!).

Birth didn't just happen to me, I triumphed over it.

As a childbirth educator for many years, I strongly encourage women to build this team around them. The more support you have for your decisions, the more likely they will become reality. In fact, even if your "dream birth" doesn't happen, these people will support you and lift you up in your time of possible disappointment or sadness.

With all the importance of these people, I fear that we occasionally forget that the most important support a woman can have for her labor doesn't actually come from without, but from within.

This is why I feel so strongly about the importance of childbirth education. So many times I hear women say things like, "I have a great midwife," or "I hired a doula," or "I trust my doctor," or "I am birthing at a birth center," as though these (excellent) choices will somehow guarantee them a great birth.

There is truth behind this thought process. You do need a birth team that you trust and you need to birth in a place and with people who are wonderful and skilled. But that is not enough if you, yourself, are not prepared.

Doulas don't feel your contractions for you.

Midwives can't make the power of birth stop so you can catch your breath.

A well trained and prepared partner cannot give you the dedication that you need.

A fabulous obstetrician cannot handle your emotional preparation for birth.

Your childbirth educator will not make you eat healthy or exercise appropriately as you prepare for birth.

All of these things women must do themselves.

In all truthfulness, I think that women have often become so accustomed to giving away their power in birth that they don't know how to take it back again. We even sometimes mistake good birth choices as some special kind of buffer that will protect us from having to dig deep and do hard work ourselves.

Frankly, this frightens the heck out of people. While truly owning your birth and preparing yourself mentally, emotionally, physically, and spiritually can be overwhelming and even a little scary, this is the most important work you can do for your birth.

When women prepare themselves as their most important

While truly owning your birth and preparing yourself mentally, emotionally, physically, and spiritually can be overwhelming and even a little scary, this is the most important work you can do for your birth.

ally for birth, they find their true power. When they own their choices and take responsibility by doing everything they can do, both in the people they surround themselves with AND with the internal and physical preparation they need, then they find real empowerment.

This is what each of us needs, but it isn't an easy road. Letting someone else "take care of us" during the vulnerable time of labor and birth is effortless. Passing the buck to professionals who know more seems like the best choice. Depending on support people to carry the burden for us sounds wonderful. But it isn't.

When women prepare themselves as their most important ally for birth, they find their true power.

Every woman deserves to leave birth a stronger woman who finally understands both her own vulnerability and her own capacity. She deserves this, but she is also the only person who can earn that feeling of triumph.

You are your most important labor support. You are strong enough to do it.

Sarah Clark is a mother of four and a childbirth educator in northern California. She has trained over 100 natural birth educators for Birth Boot Camp and loves watching women make their own birth choices. You can visit her work at www.birthbootcamp.com and www.mamabirth.blogspot.ca.

Helena Ryan

Like many of us, Helena was told all sorts of horror birth stories. She was advised to take the drugs during labor, because that was what women needed. However, Helena disagreed with the status quo, and instead surrounded herself with positive childbirth stories. She prepared using hypnobirthing, and found an incredible support person to help her through this journey. Her story is beautiful as it is a reflection of the growing number of women who are taking control of their childbirth, and of those who are determined to actually enjoy this moment in their lives.

The Birth of Cayden

"Childbirth for me was the most empowering and transformational experience of my life."

My name is Helena and I'm 33 years old. I gave birth to my first child, Cayden, on July 1st, 2014. I live in Brisbane, Australia.

When I first told people I was pregnant, nearly everyone told me horror stories of labor and how painful and difficult it is. Everyone, from strangers on the street, to colleagues and friends, would tell me to "take the drugs!" It was challenging to find positive childbirth stories and this is why my story is different.

Childbirth for me was the most empowering and transformational experience of my life. It was truly a gift and a privilege to have been able to experience the depth and range of emotions and sensations that I felt. I never knew how strong I was until those first few minutes when I held my son in my arms.

I understood that my body knew what to do, that it was designed specifically for this one job, even if it was only going to do this just once in its lifetime. Even if I didn't have a clue what to do and I had never experienced it before, I knew that if I could "get out of the way" and allow my body to birth my son, it would. I set the intention of having an empowering birthing experience where I could look back and say "that was awesome."

I chose to have a home water birth and my husband and I worked closely with my midwife from the fourth month of pregnancy. I didn't want to be in a hospital environment and work to someone else's chart, system or idea about how I should birth and in what time frame. We had experienced that 3 years earlier when my husband had cancer.

At 4 am on July 1st, 2014, my water broke and I woke up my husband. We puttered around the house for a few hours, and called my midwife to let her know. She told us that it could be hours, or it could be days, so we went about life as normal. At 8:30 am, contractions started and they were less than 5 minutes apart.

We attended hypnobirthing classes where it was described to us what contractions can feel like and how they can be different for each and every woman. I just wasn't prepared for the intensity of how they felt. They started out as cramps and quickly progressed into ripples of pressure and pain all through my back. It took my husband and me 30 minutes to realize I was actually in labor. I thought labor contractions started at the front. After 20 minutes of all the back pain on and off, we started to look up some things in "Dr. Google" and it was only then did we realize my labor had actual begun!

Within 90 minutes, my midwife, backup midwife and student midwife had all arrived. There was a mad rush to fill the pool up in time to get me in there. I dilated from 3 cm to 8 cm in under 90 minutes.

When fear is absent, there is no need for pain.

My son was posterior throughout the pregnancy, right up until the last hour before he was born, and that's why the pressure on my back was intense. I had very little resting time between contractions.

Going into a home water birth, many people asked me "what about the pain?" It never crossed my mind. When fear is absent, there is no need for pain. The contractions were painful while at the same time they were not, if that makes any sense. Once in the water, my midwife and husband encouraged me to change positions regularly to help make as much room in my pelvis as possible. The warm water helped, but my epidural that day was my husband. Justin sat at the side of the pool, and I hung onto him and wouldn't let him go. We were connected that day in a way we have never been before. I knew that if I were to get through this experience, he would be the one to get me there. I felt nothing but strength, love and calmness coming from the man I cherished. He whispered the right words in my ear, helped me move into positions, and never once let me go. As long as I had his hand, I knew I was safe and protected. He was my rock and I fell more in love with him that day than I ever thought possible.

The pushing phase for me was long and intense. It took over two hours. It was incredibly painful, beyond anything I had ever felt before. The fascinating thing about the pain, is that it isn't like a paper cut or when you stub your toe. Once a contraction ends, there is absolutely no pain or throbbing that lingers. It was very much a start and stop type of pain. There were a few times that I said aloud, "I can't do this anymore," and my midwife would tell me "you have to!" so I kept going.

The warm water helped, but my epidural that day was my husband.

As the labor began and progressed, I found myself disappearing into myself. I could hear and see what was happening around me, but couldn't connect with it. I was completely in my own space with my body and **son;** hanging onto my husband's arm and every word he said to me. Each time I said, "I can't do this," I felt myself drop even deeper into a completely peaceful space, and I was able to tap into more strength and inner-power than I even knew existed within me. Every time it was too much, I found that reserve of power within.

As a hypnobirthing mum, I watched plenty of calm and peaceful births where the mothers calmly and silently birthed away. Mine was nothing like that. With every contraction, a primal grunting and groaning would start, sometimes without me even realizing I was making it. My voice and the noise was my way of releasing the pain and energy with each contraction.

My son was born at 2:42 pm, 6 hours after the first contraction, and weighed 7lbs 4oz. He had a full head of golden hair and a true knot in his cord. He was, and is, just perfect.

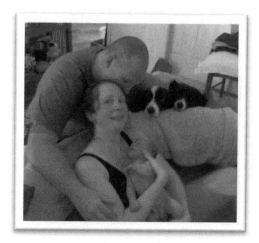

What did you like most about your childbirth experience?

Labor was like an out of body, deep experience for me. There is nothing I would have changed about it or done differently. The biggest challenge I faced with labor was the two weeks leading up to it, where I was in pre-labor the whole time. I had 6 false starts and it messed with my head. By the time my water broke, I was well and truly over being pregnant. The final months for me were also very difficult. I had to leave work early, and I was in a lot of pain.

What did you like least about your childbirth experience?

The part of labor that I cherish the most was recognizing just how strong I am as a woman and person, and just how strong my husband and I are as a couple. This strength that I've unleashed will be instrumental when I return to my business. I really believe it's made me a better wife, mother, friend and daughter. My husband played such an active role in my labor. He stepped up beyond belief. Our labor journey together has shifted, and strengthened how he sees himself as a man and husband. He hasn't been the same since, and I'm so immensely proud of him and how we walked this path together.

What would you tell an expectant mother to better prepare her for childbirth?

My advice for women who are entering this journey is to get a network around you of one or two women who have walked this path just prior to you. I found that so much time is spent being focused on the pregnancy and labor, then all of a sudden there is this little bundle in your arms and you realize you haven't spent much time learning about babies. Find someone who is willing to give advice, friendship, support, and who will allow you to cry when you need it.

The biggest piece of advice I can give is to trust yourself. Trust your intuition when it comes to everything to do with your pregnancy, labor and beyond. Trust that gut instinct when it comes to choosing the support team around you, and trust that knowingness that you get. Pregnancy and labor are just as much a spiritual journey as they are a physical journey. A mother's instinct sets in long before her baby arrives.

Trust your intuition when it comes to everything to do with your pregnancy, labor and beyond

■■

Deja' Cronley

Women are often told there is no way to guarantee the duration of labor or delivery. But why not? Why not visualize what you would like to happen? Of course fate may wish otherwise, but there is nothing wrong with anticipating something good and beautiful. This is exactly the story of Deja'. She gave birth in a loving and comfortable atmosphere, and allowed herself time to enjoy all the moments of her labor and birth. Her story brings light and positivity to the discussion surrounding childbirth.

The Birth of Scarlett

"I felt like I was high as a kite - those endorphins were amazing!"

"What is your idea of the perfect birth?" - When I read this question during my pregnancy, I envisioned the following: my labor would be on a Sunday, I would labor all day at home with my husband, watch a Dallas Cowboys football game, get in the birthing pool in the living room, and labor while overlooking the lake. I wanted a fast birth – about 3 hours. It was a nice thought...

At 38 weeks and on a Sunday morning, I got out of bed around 8:30 am, and when using the washroom, I saw discharge that looked like amniotic fluid. I took a shower, and as I was getting dressed, I felt a pop. I managed to plop on the toilet right as I gushed fluid.

Around 10:30 am, I realized I was having mild contractions about five minutes apart. I let the midwives, photographer and my parents know what was going on. The midwives said to let them know when my contractions became closer together.

I started cooking, and my husband scrubbed the house down. At 1:00 pm, the Dallas Cowboys game started, and I got on the birthing ball to watch it. I was starting to get impatient, so

I mixed clary sage essential oil with some coconut oil, and applied it to my wrist and lower abdomen, in hopes of bringing on stronger contractions.

Around 4:00 pm, my contractions were becoming more intense, but they still weren't painful. Forty five minutes later, the contractions were a bit more uncomfortable, so I texted my midwife and photographer to update them. By now it was almost 5:00 pm. I got in the shower for about twenty minutes just to relax. For the first contraction after the shower, I got on my hands and knees in the hallway, and swayed my hips. I finally felt like I was in labor!

I laid down on the blow up mattress my husband set up for me and listened to the rest of the game. My contractions were more intense but had a weird pattern: they were too close together and then nothing for about five minutes. Around 5:45 pm, I asked my husband to text the midwives to come check on me. Shortly after, my contractions went from intense to painful, so I got in the birthing tub.

Fifteen minutes later, I started moaning through contractions and all I kept thinking was, "keep my jaw loose and my moans deep to let my cervix open up". For this advice I thank you, Ina May! I asked my husband to call the midwives since they hadn't responded and they said they would send the apprentice out to check on me when they heard my moans. They weren't getting our texts and were wondering how things were going. I had my husband text the photographer and ask her to come over, and I just kept moaning and swishing my body around in the water.

I started to feel nauseous, and the next contraction I felt myself start to push. I thought I was imagining things since I had only been hurting at most an hour, so I put my finger in to check and I felt the baby's head! Shocked doesn't even begin to describe how I felt in that moment. Well, shocked and elated! I was almost done!

I got the perfect labor and perfect daughter and I can't wait to do it again!

I told my husband to tell the midwife that I could feel the baby's head an inch in. Her response was "Oh my, we're on our way." In between contractions, I looked at him and said "don't get me wrong, this hurts, but it isn't nearly as bad as I thought it would be!" A couple contractions later, the apprentice midwife showed up and she could see about a quarter of the baby's head crowning.

With that contraction I finally fully pushed – I felt the head go out then slide back in a bit. The next contraction, I pushed again and got her head halfway out, and I waited for the next contraction. While I was waiting for the next contraction (with a head halfway out of me), the other two midwives arrived, and I told them "the head is halfway out." When the next contraction finally came, I pushed and the baby shot out. She had a loose cord around her neck, so my husband and I unwrapped it, and then I brought our baby out of the water. Arms spread out, eyes wide open, and blue (very normal). I rubbed my baby's back and we heard a healthy scream and saw a nice pink color. My husband helped me out and onto the mattress. I felt like I was high as a kite – those endorphins were amazing!

After a few minutes, my husband and I figured we should look and see if the baby was a boy or girl. As I held the baby up, we realized she was a girl! I was immediately in love with Scarlett – all 6lbs 12oz of her. About 10 minutes later, the photographer arrived and got some great shots of our first hour together. I am so grateful for the 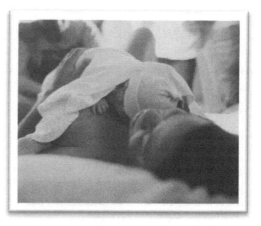 pictures we have. My husband was even sneaking pics of me in labor so I have those too!

I got exactly the birth I wanted! I went into labor on a Sunday, got to see my Cowboys play, and had a fast, but not overwhelming labor. Not only did I get the perfect labor, I also got a perfect daughter and can't wait to do it again!

What did you like most about your childbirth experience?

I loved that I got to follow my instincts and labor on my own, and in my own space with no distractions. I can't imagine hitting active labor, then having to focus on getting in the car, going to a hospital, getting checked in, having an IV started, etc., then trying to get comfortable in a foreign environment.

What did you like least about your childbirth experience?

I loved everything. My only complaint is we were unable to get the delivery videotaped by the photographer.

What would you tell an expectant mother to better prepare her for childbirth?

Do your homework and know what all of your options are. Going with the flow during labor is great, but in order to take an active part in your labor, you need to know what to expect. You need to understand what your options are, and what the pros and cons are to each suggestion you accept and choice you make.

You need to understand what your options are, and what the pros and cons are to each suggestion you accept and choice you make.

Marissa Collins

Marissa shares with us two beautiful natural water birth stories, which occurred in the comfort of her own home. She wanted to give birth peacefully and as naturally as possible. With the support of her family and doulas, Marissa got exactly the births she wanted. She felt ecstatic, and happy, and just completely overjoyed. Her birth stories show us the powerful emotions that are often present during childbirth. The mother is complete, and has given birth in a respectful and dignified manner. This is the way all births should unfold.

The Birth of Qasean Michael-Alexander Collins

"I had the most intense natural high and kept saying
"I did it, I did it!"

I was at 41 weeks on Friday, April 1st, 2011. We tried every natural way of induction possible. I was getting emotional thinking that my dreams for a home birth were not going to come true. But I knew that Qasean was going to come when he was good and ready.

My water broke at 2:53 am on Monday, April 4th. I got in the shower and had the hot water run directly on my lower back. It was like all the pressure was taken off of my back and I was able to relax in between contractions. Once I was in the tub, Roni (my doula), Laurel (her assistant) and my husband, Chris, took turns putting pressure on Bladder 31 during a contraction. This was the only thing that gave me relief from the pain.

My doula was incredible. She helped calm me, held my hand when needed, and reassured me that this was the best thing for me and baby. Chris amazed me at how attentive and supportive he was, and that he tried to do as much as he could for me. He would talk to me in between contractions or get right in front of my face and encourage me to get through it.

I loved being in the tub. During the contractions, all I could think of was Ina May Gaskin. I remember her saying that you need to relax your mouth and that would in turn relax your cervix and help with dilation. Roni wanted the baby to move lower into my pelvis so she suggested going back to the shower and it worked. After what seemed like forever to me, we transitioned back into the tub.

It was finally time to start pushing. Once I was able to concentrate on just the diaphragm, it wasn't long before I could feel his head, and then I felt his hair! The next couple contractions he was closer and closer to crowning. It was so weird and amazing that my body knew just what to do!

With the next contraction, I pushed and his head came out! I burst out laughing as I couldn't believe that I had done it! I was in such shock and awe and so excited to see him! I held him underwater and removed the cord that was partially around his neck. After the blood transferred to him from his placenta, I brought him up and onto my chest. He was covered in white vermix. I just stared at him and was lost in his beautiful little body! I stayed in the tub a little while longer until the placenta came out on its own. I had done it! All the research, videos and positive thinking paid off. I had my natural, unmedicated, home water birth! I had the most intense natural high and kept saying "I did it, I did it!" I have no idea how women do it on land…the water was amazing! Qasean Michael-Alexander was born on April 4th, 2011 at 4:30 pm.

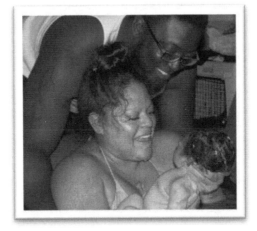

The Birth of Cataleya Elaria Jovila Collins

"I had done it once again... Such an amazing feeling."

Contractions woke me up at 4 am, and had gotten stronger around 6 am. I was still able to breathe through them, but they were becoming more intense.

Outside, I immediately smelled flowers and knew she would be named Cataleya. I ate breakfast for the extra energy I needed. By about 7:05 am, the contractions were only 7 minutes apart, and so our doula Claire came over. In between eating, I would get a contraction, and would sway with my knees bent. Claire was behind me applying pressure into my shoulders, and supporting my legs by bending and swaying with me. We were having our own little dance party in the kitchen.

I got my bathing suit top and wraparound skirt, and headed towards the tub. Once again, like with Qasean, Bladder 31 pressure point to the rescue! The hot water felt absolutely fantastic! By this time, contractions were maybe a couple minutes apart. Not soon after I was in the tub, I felt the urge to push. Chris had music playing and it was like my body was in tune with each song. It was crazy but as soon as a song would end, so would the contraction.

Claire could tell it was time to go and told me that if we were leaving for the hospital, then this was the time to go. I shook my head no. The thought of being in a car during those contractions - not going to happen. My inner animal was working – Thanks Ina May! I was very aware of where my baby was and could feel her head getting lower and lower. After a couple good pushes, she was starting to crown! I tried to relax as much as possible. I reached down, and felt a full head of hair. Once her head was out, it was a huge relief! The next contraction I had, I was able to push her out completely. During the crowning part, the music had changed to an upbeat, happy tempo, music. The kind of music that plays at the end of a happy movie. It was surreal. I

> *My inner animal was working – Thanks Ina May!*

brought her up out of the water and immediately to my chest. She was born at 9:13 am on March 7th, 2014. I had done it once again! Baby number 2 at home and in the water! Such an amazing feeling.

We hung out in the water, just enjoying the moment. Qasean woke up shortly after Cataleya was born. Once he saw the water, he wanted to go swimming. When he saw Cataleya, he had a confused, but happy face. Cataleya and I stayed in the pool until after the placenta stopped pulsating, which was quite a while after.

Cataleya latched on and nursed perfectly! Showering last time was quite difficult, but this time, it was so much easier! I then got comfy in bed, and it was time to nurse again. While nursing, Qasean came into the room with a doll, and placed it by Cataleya. That absolutely melted my heart.

We hung out in the water, just enjoying the moment.

What did you like most about your childbirth experience?

The sense of empowerment it gave me. To know that no one else touched my babies but me. It was all on my own terms, and my babies made an appearance when they wanted to!

What did you like least about your childbirth experience?

For my son, nothing. It was perfect and everything I dreamed of!

For my daughter, it was the treatment in the hospital after she was born. I felt like we were lab rats or a circus side show. Everyone had to come in, poke her, and look her over. "Ohhh look, the home birth baby!"

What would you tell an expectant mother to better prepare her for childbirth?

Be well aware of any interventions, and know what you will allow to happen. Know that birth can be amazing when you not only physically prepare (eating well and exercising), but when you also mentally prepare! If you want to go the natural birth route, then read books about it and watch videos. The more confident you are in your decision, the better the outcome will be. Say "I WILL," instead of "I'll try." Know that your body was made to birth, and trust your instincts!

Know that birth can be amazing when you not only physically prepare (eating well and exercising), but when you also mentally prepare!

Hospital Births

In many cities around the world, pregnant women have the option of giving birth in either a hospital, or in their home. For some, a hospital provides a sense of safety, and thus eases any fear they may have. For others, especially high-risk pregnancies, hospitals can provide speedy medical attention in case of any complications. There are also women who do not have the choice or the (financial) means to give birth at home, and are thus forced to give birth in a hospital. The following mothers gave birth in a hospital, and experienced both happy and sad births. Their stories contain emotions which range from extreme joy and happiness to embarrassment and anger. This is true birth, in the hospital, as experienced by the mothers themselves.

■ ■

Katherine Jubb

Katherine's birth stories show the importance of a woman's approach to childbirth. Her second birth was much more empowering for her because of the way she prepared for it, and because of how she understood it and all of its complexities. Katherine refused to be a victim, and faced birth with strong determination. She wanted to play an active role in her second birth, and thus cast herself as the main character in her story. She let birth happen, and allowed herself to be present mentally and physically. This story shows that when a woman empowers herself, she can influence her fate.

My Birth Stories

"I was not a victim. I was not trying to avoid it.
I was accepting of it and permitting it to progress."

My daughter was born after a long and grueling labor that saw me awake for 73 hours straight. Having my first baby at 21, I was about to confront an unfortunate reality. No matter how much technology there may be, how purposefully built the hospitals are, and how 'far' we think we have advanced ourselves, there is a very large disconnect between our natural biological capabilities, how women regard birth and their bodies, and how the event is managed by the health care system. While we were busy making medical advancements and inventing lifesaving technology (which is great), childbirth in the organic sense, and its ironic combination of complexity and simplicity, lost the respect and awe it deserves. Childbirth was never broken, yet someone tried to fix it as though it was flawed. As a result, now women are, on the whole, distant from and afraid of childbirth, conditioned to think of it in certain (negative) ways.

I had attended antenatal classes and I had every faith that what I was doing was right. I liked the idea of a water birth, but sometimes we don't get what we want. At midnight, leading into

Thursday, when I felt the first twinges of regular, period-like cramping, I didn't know what I should have been doing. Fuelled by curiosity, adrenaline, excitement and the 'f' word (fear), I remained awake, convinced this was happening right now! Mistake! Forty eight sleepless hours later, a trip to the hospital, and back home again, not even in established labor yet, I was beyond shattered!

By 6/7 pm on Friday evening and after yo-yoing in and out of the bath for two days and a night, I resigned to the sofa with a DVD. At about 10 pm, things felt a little more intense, and this time we went to the hospital. I was finally qualified to stay. I was at 3 cm. Only 3 cm – absolutely gutted!

I was given a TENS machine, which I loved! I labored throughout the night, entangled with wires from the TENS machine and a fetal heart monitor. After 4 hours and only one more cm dilated, they broke my waters and gave me gas-and-air to compensate for the added discomfort. I didn't know the importance of staying mobile, and had little to no energy to do much of anything anyway. The midwives in the hospital encouraged me into an all-fours position, leaning against the back of the bed. They also forced me, much against my will, off of the bed and onto a birthing ball.

I kept feeling way out of my depth and scared. I vowed she would be an only child, and I was actually utterly convinced at one point that I would die. This amuses me now, and is a testament to how little I knew about birth!

Finally, on Saturday morning at 10:22 am, when I was half asleep, I pushed my daughter into the world. Weighing 7lbs 2oz, she came to my breast. I didn't know what I was doing, and neither did she. On top of that, the support was catastrophically awful. Feeding was not established well. Her father could not stay, and I was sad to be without him.

I had wanted to birth at home, but I had an ovarian cyst, and so a hospital birth was advised.

Two years later, I was pregnant with my second baby. I started re-living in my sleep the traumatic parts of having my daughter. The details that I had since forgotten came back to me. My anxiety made me ill. I had wanted to birth at home, but I had an ovarian cyst, and so a hospital birth was advised.

The day of the birth, I went to sleep and woke at 4 am with some period-like cramping. I began the day with some extra energy, ironing dresses for my daughter and myself, and left for my antenatal appointment. When forced to sit still in the hospital, the contractions intensified. It was noon, and I was at 2.5 cm. I followed my consultant's advice, went home and had a bath. This time I discovered that I hated the TENS machine, and went back to the hospital at 3 pm.

I was at 4-5 cm now, bouncing on a birthing ball in the pool room, leaning on my partner. We were much closer this time! I drew strength and comfort from him. I had struck lucky as the midwife was really passionate about natural birth. She was quiet and reassuring. She did little and said little. I moved from the ball to the bath, and from the bath to the pool, where my entire body relaxed! I was given gas-and-air, but didn't find it helpful. However, when things were very intense, I blew into the mouth piece deeply and said to myself 'breathe the baby out,' and then breathed in regular air instead. Strange, but it worked beautifully to control and deepen my breathing, and helped keep my jaw relaxed.

My son came into the world at 5:24 pm. His cord was cut when it was no longer pulsating. The birth was so chilled out - worlds apart from my first experience! I began tandem feeding, which confused a midwife on the maternity ward, who mistakenly thought there would not be enough milk left for the little one!

With my first baby, labor happened to me. It was as if I had to suffer through it, while trying to avoid it. Yet with my second childbirth, I learned that I could interact with the process of labor and even be in control. It was happening, but not to me. I was not a victim. I was not trying to avoid it. I was accepting of it and permitting it to progress.

I learned that I could interact with the process of labor and even be in control.

I had childhood leukemia and other issues. I was used to my body failing me and causing problems, but that was irrelevant because I had just birthed a baby, with relative ease and yet enormous strength. My body and I did that! It's not a lemon after all!

My body and I did that! It's not a lemon after all!

What did you like most about your childbirth experience?

It's almost a given that the best moment is the moment you first make eye contact with the little person that has been the focus of your curiosity for the last 9 months. To finally know what they look like. To learn if they are a boy or a girl. To absorb everything about them. To hold them, touch them, and smell them. But aside from this, I enjoyed a feeling of accomplishment. The amazement at being able to get up and walk just minutes after birth. I enjoyed seeing the transformation in my partner from man to doting father.

On a scientific level, these changes that occur shortly after birth are probably associated with the euphoric high that follows birth, especially a drug-free one where hormones can act as intended. With my son, I also enjoyed all of the birth because I was more relaxed and accepting of it. I have positive memories of even the intense parts. Both births were wonderful, but they were also very different. They brought my partner and me closer together.

What did you like least about your childbirth experience?

I did not like feeling so lost, weak, afraid and out of control. During my first birth, the fear was much more intense, just like the pain. I doubt this was a coincidence! I did not like the fetal heart monitor. I did not like feeling like someone I didn't know or trust (the midwife) was in control of me. I did not like that this midwife was bossing me around when I felt weak and tired, yet I didn't know how to take responsibility myself! I did not like feeling surprised and shocked when I vomited during transition, because I had no idea this was quite normal. I did not like my stay on the maternity ward. It was not a good place to sleep!

What would you tell an expectant mother to better prepare her for childbirth?

Read about the positive side of birth. Don't just learn about the biology, about what can go wrong, and what pain relief you can have. Read positive birth stories. Attend private antenatal classes if possible, and think about employing a doula. Focus on how you can best relax during labor, as that is so important and the best tool for encouraging easy progression.

Watch birthing videos, especially home birth ones, even if you are planning a hospital birth. It's good to see birth happen away from the medical setting of a hospital, so that you can become comfortable with birth and comfortable with it being separate from a medical condition. Know that you can breathe through the intense bits. I would also highly recommend perineal massage to help avoid stitches – it worked for me!

Focus on how you can best relax during labor, as that is so important and the best tool for encouraging easy progression.

Amber Dabrowski

The following story depicts the hospital childbirth of a first time mom. Amber's due date had come and gone, and her little one was nowhere to be seen. Amber's mother had two natural births, and thus Amber understood childbirth as a natural phenomenon. She did not worry about it, but rather embraced what was happening. Unfortunately, despite feeling secure with her midwife, Amber did not appreciate the pushiness of her hospital nurse. She encourages all pregnant moms to make sure they feel comfortable and at ease during labor and delivery.

The Birth of Emmett

"I remember being in this state of emotional high…
I was so happy and so full of life."

My mother gave birth to me in a trailer down a dirt road. No lie. Yes, this was very "hippy" you would say, but thankfully my mother knew what she wanted, and knew instinctively that giving birth was natural. When I too was going to traverse this journey, I knew instinctively that giving birth was natural, and I wanted our experience to be just that: natural. I also felt it necessary to have a midwife instead of a medical doctor.

Our little boy was comfortable for a little longer than any of us anticipated but alas, the midwives at UNC were patient. I was allowed to go over my due date, and really reach a point of wanting our little boy to come. I was desperately uncomfortable and was no longer nervous about the birth.

Finally, on an early morning visit to the midwife on July 3rd (original due date was June 26th), I was dilated to 4 cm. On July 4th, I had a horrible time getting up the hill in the neighborhood. That evening, we went out for Chinese food, and I ordered something spicy, hoping to start labor. Around 9:00 pm, I started to have gas pains, which eventually turned into labor pains. I did not want to labor at the hospital too long, as I had read stories of women slowing down their labor in a hospital setting. At home, I was comfortable and in a setting that was familiar, so we stayed at home a little longer.

When I laid down, my water broke, but my contractions remained erratic. I was in so much pain that we decided to head to the hospital. Once there, we walked and stopped every time I had a contraction. We made it up to the second floor and walked into Labor and Delivery. In between contractions I signed paperwork, standing up. I laid down on the hospital bed, and had an extremely painful contraction. I was on my side, and told my husband that I felt like I had to push. My midwife told me I was at 9 cm and was ready for delivery. We were all surprised. I was wheeled immediately into the delivery room.

I was triaged as I pushed. I felt every contraction and every push. The pain of pushing a baby out is intense, yet so intense that your brain does not allow you to recognize the intensity. I felt the distinct need to push with every contraction. While pushing out our little boy, my midwife allowed me to pull up on a bar that was attached to the bed. The delivery nurse would count to ten, but there were times at the end when I could not hold out until ten.

My midwife made it clear that I was OK to stop pushing when I was ready. At one point, I was tearing up from the pain and wanting him to come out so badly. I look back now and realize just how quickly the whole birth happened. I could not prepare mentally for each step, and was left to deal with each moment I was handed. I remember just how bad the ring of fire hurt and I pushed through this. That was a bad idea, considering after the birth I had a level 3 tear. Once the ring of fire was over, I pushed out our baby's head, and I just remember how much of a physical relief that was. My midwife asked me to push when I felt another contraction, and with that, his shoulders came out.

I loved my baby boy and husband so much that I thought my heart would literally burst!

Once his shoulders were out, that was it! I reached down and pulled the rest of his body right out. Immediately, I felt this huge relief roll through my body. Emmett was then placed right on my chest at 5:05 am. I was able to give birth from start to finish in 8 hours. After the placenta was delivered, I was sewed up and stood up. From the moment Emmett was born, I was wide awake and could not go to sleep. I remember being in this state of emotional high. I loved my baby boy and husband so much that I thought my heart would literally burst! Those types of emotions only come to those of us who

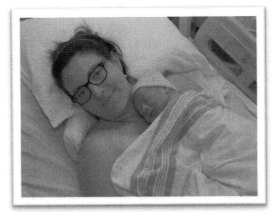

experience natural birth. I was so happy and so full of life. The whole fast-paced experience was amazing, and I am so glad I was able to have a natural childbirth.

What did you like most about your childbirth experience?

That we had a quick labor and natural childbirth. Having a balanced, respectful midwife truly helped me get through the pushing.

What did you like least about your childbirth experience?

Our labor and delivery nurse. She was so intense and pushy. Not laid back at all like our midwife.

What would you tell an expectant mother to better prepare her for childbirth?

Pick up Ina May Gaskin's book on birthing. It has so many labor and delivery stories. It was a true eye-opener of the whole experience. The most important item to know is to be relaxed and to be in a relaxing setting. If laboring at home as long as possible will help you, then do it. Also, a woman knows and understands her instinct and body better than anyone else. Go with your gut, and feel your way through the labor and delivery. The reward is so wonderful at the end!

The whole fast-paced experience was amazing, and I am so glad I was able to have a natural childbirth.

■■■

The Estimated Due Date

Lauren McClain

The first thing you want to know when you find out you're pregnant is: When will the baby be here!? When will my life change? When will I meet my sweet thing? When will I be done being pregnant?

The truth is, we can't tell you when your baby will smile, or crawl, or say "Mama," and we can't tell you when your baby will be ready to be born. Everyone is different. Not all the popcorn kernels pop at the same time, and though we can give you an ESTIMATED due date (EDD), we cannot tell you when your baby's development is ideal for birth. Only your baby can tell you that.

The estimated due date is calculated to be 280 days from the date of your last menstrual period. Doctors and midwives in the United States use Naegele's Rule. Dr. Franz Naegele practiced in 19th century Germany, and noticed that pregnancies in his practice averaged 266 days. That's 266 days from ovulation, assuming that all women have 28 day cycles and all women ovulate on day 14. We all know cycles vary, even in the same woman, and science has shown that women can ovulate anywhere between days 7-30, and even sometimes later.

Let's imagine you came off the pill right before you got pregnant. That often pushes your ovulation back, up to day 30 or even later. Your EDD will be calculated assuming you ovulated (and therefore got pregnant) on day 14. That's 16 days off. Meaning your baby isn't actually 'due' until you are 42 weeks and 2 days.

So isn't there better science for this? Something since 1820? Yes, there is. One such study from 1990 found that women of color or women who have had previous pregnancies average 269 days of pregnancy. White, first time moms averaged 274 days. The study using modern women and modern scientific processes shows we average an extra 3-8

With very few exceptions, your baby will be born when it is ready.

days. But it hasn't changed obstetrical practice. This may be in part because there have also been other studies that support the continued use of 280 days from the last menstrual period. But many women don't fit that mold.

So, if you're a first-time, white mom-to-be who knows her conception date exactly, you could need an extra 8 days tacked on to your EDD. (Just remember, when figuring conception date, that sperm can hang around waiting for an egg up to five days after sex. You don't always conceive on the day you do it, and might need to add more days!)

What about ultrasound? Embryos develop at the same rate from conception to about 10 weeks (using your handy Naegele EDD). After that, your baby will grow and develop at his own speed for the rest of his life. Ultrasounds that look at development usually aren't done until about 20 weeks, and then differ by the quality of the equipment and the skill of the clinician. The later the ultrasound, the less reliable they are for estimating development and size.

With very few exceptions, your baby will be born when it is ready. Your baby will come on his birthday. He will pick it. It can help to have a due month rather than a due date. Try not to fixate on the date given to you by Franz in 1820. You will most probably have your baby within a week either side of this date. But if you are 41 weeks pregnant, it does not mean your baby is late. It means he likes being in there and isn't ready yet.

Try not to fixate on the date given to you by Franz in 1820.

Unfortunately, it's a luxury for a baby to pick his own birthday in much of modern maternity practice. When calculating due dates, you can do your part by making sure your care provider knows if you have long cycles, and by being relaxed about your estimated due time. When people ask "when are you due?" you can just say "March" or "late June," or just tack on a few extra weeks so you get fewer "you're still pregnant?!" greetings.

Also, remember that your body needs oxytocin in large quantities to go into labor. So if you are highly anxious or upset about your baby's due date nearing or passing, you will be producing more stress hormones than anything else. No matter when you're 'due' or when other people think you are due, just relax, mama. Baby's got this.

> *No matter when you're 'due' or when other people think you are due, just relax, mama. Baby's got this.*

Lauren McClain is a childbirth educator who teaches Birth Boot Camp classes in Maryland and blogs about pregnancy, birth, and parenting at mybreechbaby.org/blog. She started the website www.mybreechbaby.org to help parents of breech babies make decisions about their care.

Mary Beth Trendos

Mary Beth, shown on our book cover, describes to us the birth of her third child, Ella. After having obstetric care for her first, Mary Beth chose midwifery care for her second and third pregnancies after realizing this care was more in line with what she wanted. Her birth story shows us that nature has a way of simplifying life at unexpected times. Mary Beth felt strong and empowered, and encourages all mothers to be active participants in their birth.

The Birth of Ella

"I've never felt so strong."

With my first pregnancy eleven years ago, I had a family doctor. She was wonderful and I was very happy with the level of care I received. Looking back, the only issue that I have is that I chose to go with a doctor for no other reason than that's what EVERYONE did. When I was expecting my second child six years later, I read up on midwifery and knew it was something I wanted to try. I had an incredible experience with them, and when I became pregnant just 14 months after having my second, I called them before I even told my husband!

The entire midwife experience encapsulates what pregnancy should be! It's a joyous, incredible, empowering journey and achievement that should be celebrated and ENJOYED, not feared.

On the day I was due with my third baby – my second daughter, I was SO excited to have a stretch and sweep done. However, there was a number of other women already in early labor, and thus the midwives preferred to not rush my birth in case none of them could attend to me. They promised that within 24 hours, someone would come out to my house to perform the sweep, and this lifted my spirits. I was ready to meet this baby!

Sure enough, the following day (Thursday, February 23rd, 2012) my midwife Ellen came to our home and checked me out. At that point. I was 1 cm dilated (the same as I had been 3 weeks earlier) and there was zero progress.

The day after my midwife visited, I found that I was losing most of my mucus plug. At lunchtime I began to have some mild contractions. By 3 pm, my contractions were still mild but consistently 4 minutes apart, and lasting about 55 – 65 seconds. We had my mom come over (with her bag just in case), and headed to meet the midwife at the hospital. As soon as we arrived, my contractions stopped and I had only one in 30 minutes. She checked me and said that my cervix was long and closed, and still only 1 cm dilated. I was quite disappointed – and embarrassed! We were sent home.

Once home, we had some dinner. By 6 pm, my contractions were bothering me enough that I went upstairs to bed and left Alex and the kids to fend for themselves. My daughter Taya came up to be with me and was unbelievably amazing; rubbing my back, asking me what I needed. I will never forget how wonderful she was, and what a crucial part of my labor she had been.

At about 7:30 pm, I decided to have a bath, since the midwives always said that it will either stop the contractions or get things moving. I was only in the bath about 10 minutes but when I got out I began to experience a lot of pain. I was leaning against the wall during contractions and had to really breathe through them. I labored alone upstairs and really tried to get myself through it. I wouldn't let myself lie down and I tried to stay relaxed through the pain to allow the baby to come down. It was excruciating but I'm so proud that I was able to do this myself.

It's a joyous, incredible, empowering journey and achievement that should be celebrated and ENJOYED, not feared.

At 8 pm the kids were in bed and I knew that things were changing for me. Thirty minutes later we got Taya out of bed, gave her the baby monitor so she could keep an eye on her sleeping brother, and we rushed to the van. Thankfully Nana pulled in the driveway as we were pulling out, and off we went to the hospital!

I was in agony on the drive. I was holding onto the handle on the ceiling of the van and the contractions were coming about a minute apart. We arrived at the hospital at 8:40 pm, I got in a wheelchair, and rushed up to the 3rd floor. As soon as we reached the L&D doors, I had another huge contraction and my water broke. I was crying in pain and I knew the baby was coming. People were telling me not to push but I had no choice!

I was rushed into the same room I'd been in earlier and was barely able to get on the bed. I could feel her head coming down. I got on the bed, and tried to take off my sweater but I only got one arm out before Ella was born! She was born at 8:48 pm, 8 minutes after arriving at the hospital! One of my favorite moments of my entire life was when she came flying out. From 1 cm at 4:30pm to delivery at 8:48 pm! All we could do was laugh and fall ridiculously in love!

Ella was beautiful and perfect at 7 pounds, 15 ounces, and 19.5 inches long. I had no tearing and no stitches. I felt wonderful! Our midwife Ellen arrived shortly after the birth and was there with us until we went home. We arrived home at 1:45 am. My mom was asleep on the couch but was very excited for us to arrive and to meet her baby granddaughter (her TENTH and final grandchild) who was only 5 hours old. When we got

home, we all went into Taya's room with Ella to wake her up so she could meet her new baby sister! It was really sweet and very special. Afterwards, Alex and I curled up in bed with our little baby girl, and fell asleep.

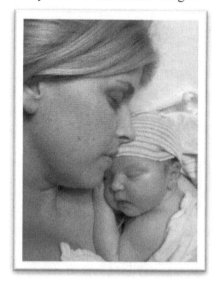

When we came downstairs the next morning, we just stared at each other in awe. We were suddenly a family of five! It was an amazing labor, an almost unbelievable delivery, and I am so grateful that I was able to have such an awesome, uncomplicated, natural birth with my baby girl! It was never my goal to do so, but it ended up being exactly what worked for me.

What did you like most about your childbirth experience?

What I liked most about my childbirth experience was how empowered I felt. My midwives were wonderful and I've never felt so strong. I was in touch with my needs and with what my body was capable of. It was amazing.

I am so grateful that I was able to have such an awesome, uncomplicated, natural birth with my baby girl!

What did you like least about your childbirth experience?

What I liked least about the experience was that my moments of not trusting in myself almost lead to me delivering my baby on the side of the road. I knew labor was progressing, but I faltered in my confidence briefly when those around me said I was likely wrong. I should have trusted myself implicitly!

What would you tell an expectant mother to better prepare her for childbirth?

The best piece of advice I can offer is to be an active participant in your birth. Be informed. Be diligent. Be insistent. This is YOUR body, YOUR baby, and YOUR delivery. Follow your instincts and make sure that whoever is in charge of your care is really listening, and has your best interests at heart. Being born is NOT a business, even though it's often treated as one.

Marika Jeziorek

This is my story of giving birth to my baby boy, Aleksander. During my pregnancy, I prepared as best as I could. I stayed fit – cycling and doing prenatal yoga and squats every single day. I kept it slow and enjoyed my time. However, after Aleksander was born, I realized that I hadn't been as prepared for childbirth as I thought I had been. I didn't know I was lacking information or resources, because I didn't even know these resources existed – they were not dispersed generously in the mainstream, to which I was accustomed to. After Aleksander was born, I became well-versed in natural and gentle childbirth and parenting, and am much better prepared for our future babies. I strongly recommend to all expectant moms that they prepare physically and mentally for this journey into motherhood. Having hope, and understanding what facilitates birth, will help tremendously. You can do it. Be strong.

The Birth of Aleksander

"We learned we had a boy, and felt incredible happiness."

I had three different EDDs. Understanding that every woman is different, I did not fret about the 'day' our baby was supposed to be born, because I knew he would be born when he was ready.

I always thought midwives were hippy-lovers who sang Kumbaya, so when I became pregnant, I knew I wanted an OB. I fell sick, and the nurse practitioner I visited at a walk-in clinic (who was also pregnant) recommended I consider midwifery care. So I began to read about the midwifery system in Ontario, and I fell in love.

As is the situation in many cities, the demand for midwifery care was huge, and completely disproportionate to the number of midwives available. I was placed on a waiting list, but having a small case of Type A personality, I called their office every other day to ask if a spot had opened up. They knew me before they even met me. And luck had it, that I almost never went to voicemail. A spot finally opened up, and I was in.

Midwifery care was and is phenomenal. Never again will I stereotypically assess a concept or method without understanding it first. My appreciation for their support has led me to always recommend this type of VIP prenatal care. And for us Ontarians, this full-time service is absolutely free, and culminates with 6 weeks of postpartum care, where you receive assistance with breastfeeding, baby-wearing, etc. Absolute bliss.

> *Midwifery care was and is phenomenal.*

I had contractions for about two days before Aleksander was born. They came and went, and I breathed through them. On April 23rd, 2013, our midwife told us that it was probably time to come check into the hospital. We arrived around 11 am, and I was 4 cm dilated. I got the room with a bathtub that I requested, and was pretty impressed with the accommodations in North Bay. My husband, Jarek, and my mom were both with me, cheering me on. Because, after all, giving birth is a big deal.

We laughed in between contractions, and focused during them. Our midwife, Audrey, was in the room, but gave us the space we enjoyed. Having tested positive for Group B Strep, I received antibiotics every so often. After a few hours, my labor stalled. Despite Audrey optimistically telling us we'd be 'done' by dinnertime, but dinnertime came and went. I labored a little in the bath tub, and walked around a few times. I preferred standing up, leaning over the bed and I remember the relief it gave me.

After a few hours, I agreed to have my waters broken, hoping it would speed things up. They never once recommended any pain relief medication, knowing I was strongly against drugs. I can't quite recall what happened next, but I do remember not remembering, or in other words, being out of it. Thus, I was probably in 'labor land.' I found myself laying on the bed (I honestly don't know how I got there), which now I know I should not have done. I should have stayed in a position that would have actually facilitated my birth, not hindered it.

After two hours of pushing, I agreed to the episiotomy, and a few minutes later, around 10 pm, our bundle of joy was born. We learned we had a boy, and felt incredible happiness. Aleksander weighed 3,290 g and was 52 cm long. Despite having a drug-free birth, it did not feel like an empowering birth. At the time, I didn't realize that an empowering birth was what I really had wanted. I knew I was missing something during my birth, but I couldn't quite identify what it was that I longed for.

After months of reflection, I now know that for our future babies, I will need to work with my body, and not against it. I will need to also dig deep and find the strength within myself. Because we all have this strength. It's just a matter of recognizing that it is within us. It is about embracing it, and taking control (as much as we can grab of it) and guiding it to the desired goal. We are mothers. We are strong.

We joked that we would give birth, and be out of the hospital 4 hours later. But then we realized how difficult it was to breastfeed. Since it was almost midnight, we decided to stay until morning. I loved having my husband stay with us, in our own private room. They provided him with his own cot, and the hospital even offered us snacks. The accommodations were simply superb – and free. The next day, we continued to practice breastfeeding, with me beeping the nurses every three hours to make sure 'I was doing it right' (we're still going strong at 19 months!) After spending another day in the hospital to get the breastfeeding help we needed, we left the following morning.

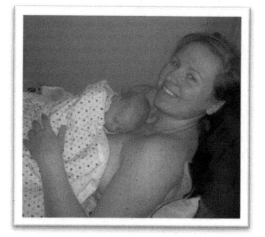

What did you like most about your childbirth experience?

I loved having my husband stay with me the entire time, even after giving birth. The hospital provided me with my own room, bathtub, and snacks. I ate freely during labor, walked around as I wanted to, and succeeded in not having any pain medication whatsoever. Success!

What did you like least about your childbirth experience?

The nurses discussing their weekend plans when I was trying to push out my baby. Not realizing that I should have stayed upright to facilitate the birth – this could have probably prevented the episiotomy. Though I could never prove it, I attribute my stalled labor to the hospital environment. Even though I loved the conditions, I did feel like I was on a schedule to deliver soon. I now know that hospitals do not equate safer or more enjoyable births (at least for low-risk pregnancies). Indeed, I hope to birth at home for our future babies.

What would you tell an expectant mother to better prepare her for childbirth?

Be positive. Approach childbirth with joy. Understand it as a normal and natural event that has been taking place since the beginning of time. However, it is also not enough to think happy thoughts. Prepare and educate yourself. By doing this, you will have the tools necessary to make decisions that will influence your birth. Work with your body, and not against it. Stay positive, ignore our cultural preference to traumatize pregnant women into thinking they need every type of intervention. Because, you most likely don't. You can do it. Remember how incredible you are, and rock your power.

> *Remember how incredible you are, and rock your power.*

Wendy S. Cruz-Chan

Wendy had wanted a natural and unmedicated childbirth in a hospital, where she would meditate peacefully in hypnosis. However, her environment and caregivers were subpar, and a series of events led to unfortunate conditions. Wendy did not have the childbirth that she longed for. She did not feel in control, or empowered. She recognizes the need to feel confident and good when giving birth, and encourages all expectant moms to consider where and how they give birth.

The Birth of Ariya

"I held her for the first time, as I wept,
feeling pure love and happiness"

On November 3rd, 2011, I woke up at 3:05 am feeling mild cramps. I was already at 38 weeks' gestation, so I naturally assumed that it was Braxton Hicks contractions. My husband John was studying for his finals at his parents' place in Queens, New York, leaving me home with my family. I was feeling the rushes come every 6-7 minutes. They were generally mild, so I went back to sleep, thinking nothing of them. By 5 am, I could no longer sleep because the rushes were getting stronger. I took a warm shower, had a bowl of cereal, and then sat down on my bed to catch up on my baby reading. Moments later, I felt a small gush of warm liquid between my legs. I thought to myself "Is this it? My water breaking?" I put on a pad and went to my mother's room to wake her up. I called John at 6:30 am, telling him my water broke, and that I was getting ready to go to the hospital with my mother. I was feeling excited, anxious, and scared at the same time since it was my first birth.

While in the taxi with my mother, it felt as though every bump we hit on the road increased the intensity of my contractions. I tried to concentrate on listening to the morning radio and on ignoring the pain. At 8 am, we had finally arrived at the hospital. I climbed out of the taxi, took four steps towards the hospital, and suddenly I knew what it meant to experience Niagara Falls. My mother and I laughed so hard. I waddled into the emergency entrance while putting pressure on my vagina, hoping it would help to slow down the flow of my water breaking. Once inside, I got wheeled up to the Labor & Delivery floor, where I found John waiting for me.

I changed into my ugly and uncomfortable hospital gown as I was instructed, after which the attending nurse put an IV in me and told me to sign my life away on their consent form. I hesitated. I was so scared of the types of medication they would give me; but I didn't have the energy to argue or fight with them. I did what they asked me to do. After the doctor examined me, I was 3 cm dilated and indeed in labor.

I requested the lights to be turned off and everyone to be quiet as I tried to meditate with the hypnobirthing soundtrack on my iPod. At 11 am, my husband John informed me that one of the nurses thought I was selfish to have such a request. To say that I felt my blood boiling is an understatement, and I lost my concentration at 6 cm dilated. Me?! Selfish?! Of course I was, I was in labor! I got mad and told the head nurse that I didn't want that particular nurse to attend to me. I was so upset I could not go back into my relaxed state, and my labor became stalled for two hours in the same dilation. As a result, my nurse gave me Pitocin and the real fun had begun. I developed a high fever due to the doctors checking my vagina at the top of every hour, causing me to contract a bacteria. My doctor came in and told me I had to get an epidural to control my fever and pain. It broke my heart because I was really set on having a natural birth. At that moment, I felt I had no choice but to agree.

At 1 pm, I was fully immersed in the effects of the epidural and some other drugs they had given me for my fever, plus medicine for the nausea, and fell asleep. Sometime after 4:30 pm, I was 9 cm dilated and the epidural was wearing off. I was moaning in pain. I found moaning very helpful as I was going through my contractions. I saw nurses

I found moaning very helpful as I was going through my contractions.

setting up my delivery room with equipment for the arrival of my baby.

By 5:30 pm, I was fully alert and overwhelmed by the pressure and pain of my contractions. All of a sudden, I felt a sharp, stabbing pain in my lower left side of my back, so I screamed and panicked. My mother at my right side held my hand as I looked into her eyes, crying. I told her I'm not ready yet, and that I'm too scared to push. John was at my left side giving me loving and encouraging words as the realization of needing to push came over me. The doctor rushed to the front of me and told me to push. John and my mother counted to 10 as I bared down with all my might. With each contraction, the doctor told me to push to help my baby descend down my birth canal. I remembered I had packed a hand-held mirror and told my mother to hold it for me at an angle so I could see my baby's head.

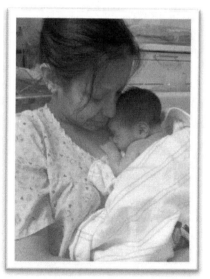

At that moment I was greeted with the site of a wrinkled scalp and my baby's dark hair. I had forgotten all about the pain I was feeling and just pushed. At 5:56 pm, my daughter Ariya was born, weighing in at 6 pounds and 12 ounces. They put her on my chest right away and I held her for the first time, as I wept, feeling pure love and happiness. My baby girl was finally here.

What did you like most about your childbirth experience?

The only part I enjoyed was when I was meditating, during the first phase of my labor. I was at peace and felt in control of my body.

What did you like least about your childbirth experience?

What I liked least about my childbirth experience was that rude nurse who told my husband that I was being selfish by wanting peace and quiet in my labor room. Also, when I was developing a fever, I really did not want any medical intervention at all. It killed my dream of having a natural birth.

What would you tell an expectant mother to better prepare her for childbirth?

If an expectant mom is told that she is a low-risk pregnant woman, then I would encourage her to explore her options of a natural childbirth outside of a hospital. Whether she wants to have a home birth, a water birth, or to birth in a birthing center, she has the power and the right to choose how and where she gives birth.

Whether she wants to have a home birth, a water birth, or to birth in a birthing center, she has the power and the right to choose how and where she gives birth.

Preparing For a Natural Hospital Birth

Sarah Clark

Is it possible to have a natural birth in the hospital? Of course it is! There is a lot of talk in the natural birth community about home birth and how fantastic it is. I am, of course, a fan of home birth. But realistically, most women will be birthing in the hospital for whatever reason. It IS possible to have a good, enjoyable, and natural birth in the hospital but there are some things that can make it more likely. Let's talk about some ways to ensure that you get a natural birth in the hospital.

RULE 1- YOUR CHOICE OF HOSPITAL IS VERY IMPORTANT IF YOU WANT A NATURAL HOSPITAL BIRTH.

You need to be very aware of the hospital policies where you will be birthing. If your hospital has rules that make it very difficult to have a natural birth, then you may want to shop around for another one. The following is a list of hospital rules and policies that work against natural birth:

- Constant monitoring (as opposed to intermittent)
- Mandatory IV (as opposed to only needed if medicated, and at the very least, a hep lock should be available)
- Supine positions required, for laboring and pushing
- Standard breaking of the bag of water
- Heavy pressure to induce labor by 40 weeks
- A strict NPO (nothing by mouth) policy (are you allowed to eat in labor?)

Other things you will want to check into:

- What is your hospital's C-section rate? (You can find them listed by state at "The Unnecesarean")
- What is your care provider's C-section rate?
- What is the induction rate?
- What is the epidural rate?
- What is their policy on walking around?

- How do they feel about doulas?
- Do they have midwives on staff?

Here is the thing: please be honest with yourself about these factors. I have seen women "say" they want a natural birth and then choose to birth at a hospital that is literally the WORST in the entire state, simply because it was convenient for them to drive to.

The chances of you not making it to the hospital in time to have your baby are very slim, especially for a first-time mother. If you are not willing to drive a little way in order to birth in a hospital that is respectful of your wishes, then you may not have the natural birth that (you say) you want.

Yes, it is possible to birth naturally in a hostile environment. It just won't be easy, and you will probably have to fight. Do you really want to fight while you are in labor?

RULE 2- CHOOSE YOUR CARE PROVIDER CAREFULLY

The next most important thing when planning a natural hospital birth is how your care provider feels about natural birth. Personally, I am a big fan of midwifery care. If your hospital has no midwives on staff, then that says something very powerful about how they view birth. Namely, it says they view it as pathological.

I have lived by many hospitals that have midwives on staff. In fact, there are a few in my area in which ALL women are assigned a midwife and only see an OB if they become high risk. Midwives are going to be trained more heavily in the normality of birth, and will transfer care if they find that there is a need.

There is this thought that midwife = home birth or midwife = no medical training. Neither is true. Yes, there are midwives who are only home birth midwives. But a hospital-based midwife is going to be a CNM, a certified nurse midwife. That means (usually) that she is an RN that has an advanced degree specializing in midwifery. These women often are very good at what they do. Yes, sometimes they are a little more medically minded than your typical home birth midwife. But, if you want to birth in the hospital, then that is your midwifery option.

So, go with a midwife if you can. If an OB is your only option, then ask them the same questions as above. Take in your birth plan. Go over it with them. Find out what works and what doesn't. Be realistic and ask hard questions. Do not be brushed off. If you are, then CHANGE PROVIDERS. You are paying for this, so don't pay for something that you do not want.

RULE 3 - TAKE A GOOD BIRTH PREP CLASS

A good birth class can really help you prepare for your natural hospital birth. It should include the following:

- An overview of the birth process
- Training of your birth partner (husband, wife, etc.)
- Relaxation training (so that you can avoid medications)
- An overview of various interventions, when they are needed, and how to avoid them if not needed
- Postpartum preparations
- Learning to communicate with your birth team

I help with Birth Boot Camp, where we prepare the partner as best as we can. Whichever class you choose, the longer the birth class, the more it will help. And be sure to take a class that is independent of the hospital. Many hospital classes tend to be more focused on teaching you how to be a good patient rather than how to have a natural birth.

A well prepared partner will really make your life easier. Think about how tense YOU will be if your partner is scared to death because he doesn't know what is going on and is freaked that you are moaning in public. Prepare him too.

Reading, preparing yourself, and practicing relaxation outside of class is wonderfully helpful too.

RULE 4- THINK ABOUT A DOULA

Doulas are not for everybody, but they can really help both mom and dad have a better hospital birth. Even when you have prepared well for a birth class, a doula can help you remember what you have learned. Even lots of dads just rave about their doula. If you want your partner to be your main source of comfort, you can always talk to the doula about helping HIM, help you. Labor can be long and an extra pair of hands can be really helpful.

Labor can be long and an extra pair of hands can be really helpful.

EXTRA TIPS

Some other helpful tips include:

- Do not arrive at your birth place too early. I am not going to tell you not to go to the hospital. If you want to go, then go. But many women cite the fact that they labored mostly at HOME as the reason why they were able to have a natural hospital birth.
- Where are you comfortable and where can you most labor how you want? Induction agents are so commonly used today, even for women already in labor. If you want to avoid them, then you may want to get some of your dilation out of the way at home, where you can move freely.
- Eat well during pregnancy so that you are low risk. Check out the Brewer Diet and consider following it. Your health pre-pregnancy may be important too. Taking better care of yourself can help you have the birth you want.

Natural hospital births are possible, but they require work and commitment. You can do it!

Sarah Clark is a mother of four and a childbirth educator in northern California. She has trained over 100 natural birth educators for Birth Boot Camp and loves watching women make their own birth choices. You can visit her work at www.birthbootcamp.com and www.mamabirth.blogspot.ca.

Hazel Woodward

Because of a medical complication that made itself evident during her pregnancy, Hazel learned that she would need to deliver her baby in a hospital. She remained positive, and was accepting of this fate. What is so humbly surprising in her story, is that even when her plan was being bulldozed through, Hazel considered the other women laboring nearby, and acted in a way as to not worry them. Her story is a prime example of how women can care so deeply for other women, even when they are in such a transitional stage as labor and delivery.

Completion: The Birth of Michael Bailey

*"But in time, my heart, as well as my head, understood that what
I did was what was right and safe for my baby,
and it had to be that way."*

Every evening (or as many as possible) I look to the sky, with reverence, to find the prettiest piece. When I find it I smile, for that is where she is now, my Mother, looking down on me, hopefully proud of me, giving me strength. This night was no different. I may have been alone, in a hospital ward, in labor, but I was OK. The person I needed to be with me, was with me.

I am Hazel Woodward. I was 32 when I gave birth to my beautiful son Michael Bailey in 2011, in Merseyside, England. During my pregnancy I learned that my baby would be big, 10lbs or more, and that I was carrying excess water (polyhydramnios). As a result, my risk was upgraded to high.

I was determined that my birth would be as natural as I could bear, with as little intervention as possible. I wanted skin to skin, to use a TENS machine, and to play music to relax me. I read books about natural childbirth, and I mentally prepared myself for the experience.

I was 39+6 when I awoke at 4 am to the feeling of baby flailing and thrashing around like a little fishy. I knew something was happening. I sat up and felt some water leak out. It wasn't the gush I had been prepared for, but I was fairly certain that my waters had broken. I felt calm, very calm. It wasn't the painful, mad dash that TV and movies would have you believe! Once we got to the hospital, I was monitored, and baby was fine. They told me I was having contractions, but I couldn't feel them yet. I was advised to stay on the ward to be monitored, but, as it was 5 am and visiting time only began at 8 am, my husband would have to leave and return later.

At 8 am, my husband arrived and we sat reading the papers and watching TV all day. I felt no contractions. I spent 28 hours after my waters had broken waiting to feel contractions. By 8 am the following day, I knew I was in labor! I had had a bath that provided great pain relief, and when I got out, I felt awful. I was at 4 cm, with contractions coming every 4 minutes. Once in the delivery room, I was using a TENS machine to control the pain, and found it was a good distraction, pressing the various buttons. I was told baby was in distress and that they might need to deliver him fast by caesarean section. The pain that I had been successfully managing now went through the roof. I was crying and very upset as they conferred with the doctor. The decision was made that I needed to have a caesarean, and I was devastated.

I had had a bath that provided great pain relief.

I had blood taken, and changed into a gown. I had to sign forms and decide whether to be put to sleep or stay awake, in which case my husband could come to watch. I decided on the latter, and I was wheeled down to theatre trying to stifle my tears, as I didn't want to worry other mums-to-be.

When we arrived at the theatre, it was like a movie set. There were at least 10 people bustling around, preparing. There were massive lights up. I was dumbfounded. I was talked through the process and what was happening. I bent over a pillow and the anesthetist gave me an injection before administering the spinal block. I had to stop him while I had a contraction, because you have to stay very still, and I was told that would be the last contraction I would feel. It was. My legs tingled but soon I had no feeling whatsoever. A sheet was erected and I heard the surgeons discuss the first incision. My husband arrived and we tensely awaited the arrival of our baby.

Pediatricians were assembled ready to check baby over. I was warned I would feel pressure, and then baby came out. He was rushed off and it felt like the longest time before he cried. When he did, tears rolled down my face.

The first time I set eyes on my baby, I fell in love. He was perfect. He had dark hair and weighed 8lbs 9oz, nowhere near the 10lb baby they told us to expect. But I only had a glance as he had to be rushed off to the Special Care Baby Unit (SCBU). I went down to recovery for half an hour, and when I returned to the ward, my husband was there with a photo of our baby. He was being treated for possible sepsis. That evening my husband went to visit him and as I had wished, he was the first to hold him.

My son and I stayed a week at the hospital, where I spent as much time with him as possible. I nearly ran out of the hospital the day we were discharged. I was told he was perfectly healthy, and to treat him like a normal baby.

We managed to establish breastfeeding, despite tongue tie and other setbacks, and successfully continued for 20 months. Breastfeeding strengthened our bond, which I felt was jeopardized after our traumatic birth and separation.

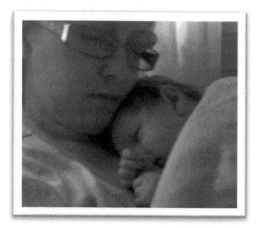

I often cried, when I was alone, because I felt robbed of the natural childbirth experience I had planned. But in time, my heart, as well as my head, understood that what I did was what was right and safe for my baby, and it had to be that way. I got through it with a strength that my mother gave me and I'm sure she would be so proud of her grandson. Having my son has made me understand her and feel closer to her than ever.

What did you like most about your childbirth experience?

My childbirth experience made me realize how strong I am; how I can hold it together when I need to; and how my body is amazing as it can carry and fully sustain a baby for so long.

What did you like least about your childbirth experience?

I least liked the fear I felt in the moments when I realized that I would have to experience the highest level of medical intervention, and the pain that it caused due to my stress levels increasing.

What would you tell an expectant mother to better prepare her for childbirth?

I would tell any expectant mother to be open minded and flexible about your birth experience. It does not make you a failure if your labor does not go the way you had planned. Sometimes Mother Nature throws in some surprises! But if she does, all is not lost; you can still bond with your baby. You may still be able to establish breastfeeding should you wish to, no matter what obstacles are thrown your way. The last piece of advice I would give, is to accept the help you need.

Be open minded and flexible about your birth experience.

Heather Jarrett

Heather wanted to deliver her baby in the most natural way possible, but accepted the possibility that her childbirth may not go according to plan. A condition during her third trimester had a snowball effect on her labor and delivery, which did not happen as she had hoped. Despite the result, Heather was content with how she stayed true to her goals as much as she could, even in the wake of very troubling circumstances. She holds no resentment, and instead continues to embrace childbirth as a natural phenomenon that may or may not need medical intervention. Even though she did not have the birth she wanted, Heather maintains a great attitude towards this remarkable milestone, and continues to encourage other women to seek out as positive and as natural of a childbirth as possible.

The Birth of Caleb John

"But most of all, just try to relax and enjoy everything..."

My first pregnancy was spent doing yoga, visualization, meditation, sitting on a birth ball, and attending a holistic pregnancy and birth group. I wanted an unmedicated home water birth with a midwife and doula. I would initiate breastfeeding right away, delay cord clamping, and have my placenta encapsulated. I didn't want to be so stuck on my 'ideal' that I neglected to consider the possibility of something going wrong, so I tried to prepare for other outcomes as well.

At 31 weeks, I felt a trickle of fluid. A midwife at my local hospital shrugged it off, saying it was probably just watery cervical mucus. I'm still upset that she didn't test for amniotic fluid. The next two days, the fluid would continue to trickle out. I decided to go to the hospital then, instead of waiting. The doctor did a vaginal exam, and a huge gush of fluid came out. My water had broken, and I burst into tears. She explained what would happen, including the risks of Preterm Premature Rupture of Membranes (PPROM).

The midwives said I didn't need to be on bed rest, but I felt differently. I was hoping to make it to at least 34 weeks. My first outpatient appointment was the next day, and my white cells were slightly elevated. The midwife attributed that to the treatment I'd had, rather than to an infection.

One night, I had the biggest gush of waters I'd ever had. I called the hospital but the midwife said it was normal for PPROM. I felt this was a warning my body would soon go into labor. The next night, my contractions got stronger, and the amniotic fluid had also gotten darker and smellier - signs of infection. I called the hospital and they advised me to come in.

My contractions were 5 minutes apart, and the fetal monitor picked them up. The doctor confirmed infection had set in and advised labor was the best course of action. I was 32 weeks + 3days. We called our doula, and were shown to a delivery suite. I was put on an IV and antibiotics, told to lie on the bed, and was hooked up to a monitor. My birth plan was dissolving before my eyes. I felt helpless.

The next hour, several staff members came to speak with us, which stressed me out so much that my contractions stopped. When my doula arrived, we tried everything to get my labor going again. The doctor had already mentioned Syntocinon, which I declined.

While I was trying to stimulate contractions, the midwife came in every 15 minutes to check the monitor. She told me the baby's heart rate wasn't being picked up because of my position. I felt pressured to lay still on the bed so the monitor could do its job - even though I wouldn't be free to do mine! It was impossible to get into labor with the constant interruptions. The doctor came back to suggest Syntocinon again. I declined. I was not dilated at all, but was effacing. I still felt very calm at this point.

I went for a walk outside to get my contractions going, and they did. Once back in the delivery suite, I found a position that intensified the rushes. It felt

Once back in the delivery suite, I found a position that intensified the rushes. It felt amazing, and I wanted to keep going.

amazing, and I wanted to keep going. Unfortunately, the midwife came in again and told me that they weren't "real" contractions since they weren't being picked up by the monitor.

The doctor suggested augmentation again. I felt it was inevitable to have it because the midwife and doctor wouldn't leave me alone long enough to get into labor on my own. After being offered it seven times, the Syntocinon was finally started on the lowest dose. I was told to lie still in bed so the monitor could pick up baby's heart rate. The next three hours the dose was increased six times, but I didn't have a single contraction.

My temperature had gone up slightly and the baby's heart rate had dropped a bit. I knew what was coming. I consented to the C-section. I went numb and wouldn't look at anyone. Half an hour later I was sitting on the operating table.

The anesthetist tried placing the spinal three times. It was incredibly painful. A second anesthetist came in, and he got it on the first attempt. I knew I was being cut, and I could feel a lot of vigorous pushing, but there was no pain. A few minutes later, Caleb John was born at 6:25 pm, weighing 4lbs 10oz. As soon as I heard his cry, tears welled in my eyes.

My wonder and elation was short-lived. They cut Caleb's cord right away, gave him some oxygen, and took him to SCBU. I laid on the table and was stitched back up. The consultant said that although our baby needed a bit of help breathing, he was otherwise healthy. Eventually, I was taken to him. I wasn't allowed to hold him so I had to settle for touching him through the holes in the incubator. Afterwards, I was taken to what would be my room for the next five days.

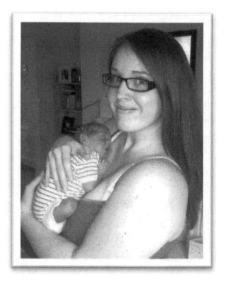

My room wasn't designed for couples, so

I was alone each night. My first night as a mother, our first night as a family, was spent apart with two of us in the hospital. Even though I knew my baby was fine, I couldn't check on him and it was the worst feeling in the world. Everything felt very wrong, and the separation was so painful.

I was traumatized by the labor and delivery, and by the weeks Caleb had to spend in the hospital. I missed out on so much. That is time I can never have back. I didn't get to hold my son until he was 15 hours old; I wasn't alone with him until he was 2 weeks old. The staff wouldn't 'let' me breastfeed him initially (I ignored them and did it anyway). I completely missed that bonding time with him right after birth, and I was not the first person to touch or hold him, bathe him, or feed him. Until he came home 18 days later, I didn't feel like he was really mine.

What did you like most about your childbirth experience?

The support from my doula. I loved that my partner and I stayed true to our beliefs as much as we could, that my baby lived, and that he was remarkably healthy for a preemie.

I loved that my partner and I stayed true to our beliefs as much as we could, that my baby lived, and that he was remarkably healthy for a preemie.

What did you like least about your childbirth experience?

Everything else! The pressure from staff, the environment, the constant interference and undermining of what I felt, the awful botched attempts at a spinal, the ensuing spinal migraines and epidural blood patch to fix them, having to stay apart from my baby, not being able to hold him or see him. I still struggle to think about it all.

What would you tell an expectant mother to better prepare her for childbirth?

Find a good doula. Read only positive things about childbirth, such as Ina May's "Guide to Childbirth." Know your rights and the local laws and guidelines. Contact your local La Leche League before you give birth so you know who to contact if you experience problems with breastfeeding in the first few days (or after). Learn how to be your own advocate, and your baby's advocate. But most of all, just try to relax and enjoy everything.

Learn how to be your own advocate, and your baby's advocate.

Katie Sorenson

Katie had wanted a natural birth with the help of hypnosis and the support of a doula. She felt well prepared for birth, and felt content with what was about to happen. However, when things took a turn, she gave birth differently than she had expected. She encourages all expectant moms to prepare for a positive birth, and to feel in control during this incredible time. Katie also mentions a very important postpartum reality that is often hushed, but that deserves our full attention.

The Birth of Evan Rees Sorenson

"I looked forward to giving birth, and felt calm and confident."

My story begins early in my pregnancy when I looked into having a doula attend my birth. I found an amazing doula, Ricky, who also introduced me to the wonderful world of hypnobabies. I decided I wanted to use the power of hypnosis to bring my baby into this world.

My guess date was February 11th, but my baby had other plans. I started having pressure waves at 3:00 am on January 25th. They seemed to progress, but then stopped for a while around 6:00 am. The waves started again at 9:00 am and were about 15 minutes apart, eventually increasing in intensity and frequency. My mother-in-law came over to take some pregnancy photos that afternoon, and she let me know that this was probably it! I went about my day, but was eventually ready for some extra support and wanted Ricky to come. By 4:30 pm, my waves were getting more intense. They were lasting a minute and coming every three minutes. We decided it was time to head to the hospital and let Ricky know to meet us there.

I arrived at the hospital at 5:45 pm. The nurse checked me and I was somewhere between 5 and 7 cm dilated. I started feeling a bit nauseous at this point. Ricky had some peppermint essential oil that really helped. At 6:30 pm, I hit the shower.

Jordan aimed the spray on my back and Ricky was giving me birth prompts through every wave to help me stay focused on my hypnosis.

I came out of the tub at 7:30 pm, and moved onto the bed into a hands and knees position, after which I started listening to "Birth Guide – Easy First Stage".

Things started to get more intense around 8:15 pm and the shakes kicked in. It seemed that I was entering into transition. I continued to chant "Peace", "Open" and "Blue" (which was the color I envisioned my "hypno-anesthesia" to be) through my pressure waves. I needed to be in a hands and knees position during every wave though, so I could only rest on my side in between.

I continued to chant "Peace", "Open" and "Blue" through my pressure waves.

The doctor checked me at 11:30 pm and I was 9.5 cm dilated, with a slight anterior lip. She offered to break my water, but I wasn't interested. I headed back to the refuge of the dark bathroom and found that what worked best was sitting backwards on the toilet during the wave, and then standing and rocking in between the waves.

By 2:30 am, I was ready to be back in the bed again. I was so exhausted by this point. I even started chanting "Out" trying to encourage baby to come out. After another hour had passed, my nurse suggested that I have my water broken. I still wasn't too sure. At 4:30 am, I decided to have it done. The fluid was clear and I was fully dilated. Around 6:00 am I experienced some more nausea, and started to actively push a little more instead of just breathing baby down.

At 8:30 am, the doctor came in and checked me. She found baby to be in the posterior position, which is likely what was holding things up. She recommended that I consider having an epidural to increase my chances of having a vaginal birth, and to rotate the baby around. Though we had wanted to avoid an epidural and had come so far without any medical intervention, I wanted to give myself the best chance at having a vaginal birth, so we agreed. The epidural was placed at 9:30 am and I was feeling relief ten minutes later. At 11:45 am, baby was still posterior, but had come down slightly. The doctor had me move into a different position to try and help baby rotate around. Ricky kept giving me doses of a homeopathic remedy to turn baby and I listened to the "Turn Posterior Baby" hypnosis track.

At 1:00 pm, the baby still hadn't turned around. The doctor tried to turn baby manually but wasn't able to. She suggested that I be augmented with oxytocin to strengthen the pressure waves and to help baby turn. I rested on and off and the oxytocin was started at 2:00 pm.

At 3:00 pm, a new OB came in to talk to us. I had spiked a fever so she suggested antibiotics. She also suggested a C-section and explained her reasoning thoroughly. For whatever reason, baby was not rotating to an anterior position and it was very clear that he wasn't coming out the natural way in the position he was in. We decided to go ahead with it as we believed that it was the best choice for baby and me.

At 3:35 pm, I was taken to the OR to have my baby. Once Evan was born they whisked him away so the nurses could give him a good once over. Jordan and Evan were then transferred to another room, while they put me to sleep to be stitched up. Proud papa held his new son, skin to skin on his chest, and took him all in. After a while, he was given a bath in the nursery while Jordan looked on. Once I came out of recovery, I was brought to my room and was finally able to meet my little prince and hold my son for the first time.

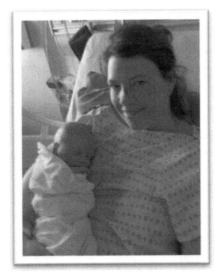

What did you like most about your childbirth experience?

Although my birth did not go at all
according to plan, it was still an amazing
experience. Looking back, I'm so happy I
chose to use hypnobabies and a hypno-
supportive doula. This is what I liked
most about my birthing experience.
Hypnobabies allowed me to feel in
control of my birth and my body.

*I'm so happy I
chose to use
hypnobabies
and a hypno-
supportive
doula.*

What did you like least about your childbirth experience?

My C-section was the least enjoyable part of my birth. I was glad
that I had read about it and knew what to expect, but I was not
prepared for the long recovery and pain that came with the major
surgery. I was also not prepared for the sense of loss I would feel
at not having a vaginal birth. It was devastating to me at the
time, but now I have made peace with it.

**What would you tell an expectant mother to better prepare
her for childbirth?**

To expectant mothers out there reading my story, don't be
frightened by my long birthing process or outcome. Trust your
body. Trust your baby. If you are hoping to have a natural birth,
look into the hypnobabies program. Before hypnobabies, I was
terrified to give birth. Once I began to experience and practice it,
I looked forward to giving birth, and felt calm and confident.

When preparing for a hospital birth, pack enough supplies for a
3-5 day stay, you never know what path your birth may take, and
it is much better to have more of everything you need.

Don't be surprised if you feel extremely emotional, weepy and
disconnected from baby around days 3-5 after giving birth. The

Baby Blues is an awful event that doesn't affect everyone. I had heard about them but no one warned me how awful it could be. It shocked me and made me feel like a horrible person. Now, I make it a point to mention it to any of my pregnant friends. Your hormones are doing crazy things and it's completely normal!

I had my placenta encapsulated and as soon as I started taking these pills I felt better and more like myself. If you do experience this and it doesn't pass after a few weeks, don't be afraid to talk to your doctor. Postpartum depression is nothing to be ashamed of and it's not in your control, but getting help and support is!

Postpartum depression is nothing to be ashamed of and it's not in your control, but getting help and support is!

Breech Babies

By Lauren McClain

You probably know someone who had a breech baby, and she probably had a caesarean. Though breech position is unusual (about 4% of term pregnancies), it is not rare. Many women get caught at the end of pregnancy with a surprise breech and do not have much time to figure out what to do about it. Without information, many women find they do not have any options. Learning some basics about breech birth ahead of time can save you a lot of anxiety and hassle in case you discover a breech at the end of your pregnancy. A caesarean is usually not necessary.

Having a breech baby throws you into a decision-making circus. Do you try to turn the baby? How do you give birth? Should you try an external cephalic version for breech (ECV)? Which of the myriad methods for turning will you pursue? How much time should you spend trying to turn the baby? How much money? When do you stop trying? For when should you schedule a planned caesarean? How far are you willing to travel for a vaginal birth attended by a skilled caregiver? If you cannot find someone, how about unattended childbirth for breech? How do you interpret the conflicting studies you keep reading about? All of this uncertainty is stressful. Here are some of the issues you should be aware of as soon as possible in any pregnancy.

AVOIDING A MALPOSITIONED OR BREECH BABY

No one really knows why babies are breech. There are some factors we strongly suspect are involved, but if you have a breech baby at term, it is very likely you will never know why. And that's OK.

You can often encourage optimal fetal positioning by having good posture and doing exercises in pregnancy. Keeping well aligned, strong and supple in the pelvic area will help baby get in the best position for birth. Excessive sitting and asymmetric postures and movements are all linked to breech pregnancies. Sofas, recliners, and bucket seats (like in a car) are notoriously bad for baby's position. Midwives who work among the Amish noted a significant increase in breech babies when their communities switched from using only hard chairs to using couches and recliners. Chiropractic care can help you maintain balance in your pelvis and uterine fascia and ligaments, making breech less likely.

WHEN TO CHECK FOR A BREECH BABY

The majority of babies turn and stay head down between 28-32 weeks. You should ask your caregiver what position your baby is in at 32 weeks. If you feel a round ball that you can wobble on the top of your belly, it's likely a head. Most obstetricians do not check the baby's position (or do not tell you about it) until 36 weeks.

TURNING YOUR BABY

You may feel that your baby is breech for a reason, and you may not want to turn your baby. Babies do know how to be born breech. There are some amazing videos[1] of the instinctual birthing movements of babies born feet or butt first. Breech babies do encounter problems on the way out more often, though, so if you feel inclined, there are many, many ways people have claimed success in turning breech babies.[2] Many can be done by you at no cost and at no risk. Doing inversions and the breech tilt, hypnotherapy, homeopathy, and chiropractic care can all turn a breech baby. You can even turn a breech baby with essential oils.

Interestingly, women who plan a vaginal breech birth have babies who turn head-down spontaneously twice as often as women who plan a caesarean. This may be due to the lower-level of stress these mothers have, thinking of their baby as a variation of normal instead of a problem to be dealt with.

---

[1] https://www.youtube.com/watch?v=jD5939e5PZ8
[2] http://www.mybreechbaby.org/breech-turning-techniques.html

VAGINAL BREECH BIRTH

Recent research[3] shows that vaginal breech birth is just as safe as or safer than caesarean breech birth for the baby. Vaginal birth is almost always safer for mom and always safer for the mother's subsequent babies. The American and Canadian OB groups (ACOG and SOCG) recommend vaginal breech birth in select cases. One of the cases is that you have an OB who is experienced and confident in breech delivery.

Unfortunately, due in part to a flawed study[4] released in 2000, and a history of insurance companies threatening teaching hospitals that taught breech skills, most caregivers today have had no opportunity to practice vaginal breech birth. The study was debunked around 2006, but so few people now remember how to attend a vaginal breech, or simply don't want to. Though studies continue to be conducted, the results tend to depend on the skill of the attendants. Michael Odent, one of the leading mother-baby friendly obstetricians in the world says, "Breech birth by people who are afraid of breech birth is very dangerous." This is largely because of rough or hasty handling of a partly-born baby.

You may have heard the phrase "Hands off the breech!"[5] Practitioners have found that breech babies know how to be born and that by letting them birth themselves, they come out safer. Unless the head becomes entrapped, many breech-friendly practitioners will keep their hands off the breech. These experiences have also taught us that women birthing instinctively also know how to birth breech babies, and, if in tune with their body, will move in such a way as to facilitate the easiest birth.

CESAREAN BREECH BIRTH

A little known fact is that a caesarean does not remove all the danger of breech birth. It is safer to come out head-first,

---

[3] http://www.mybreechbaby.org/safety-of-vaginal-breech-birth.html
[4] http://www.mybreechbaby.org/term-breech-trial1.html
[5] http://www.aims.org.uk/Journal/Vol10No3/handOffbreech.htm

no matter whether it is an abdominal or vaginal delivery. Your baby still has to be squeezed and maneuvered out of a small hole; it is just quicker and more managed with a caesarean. Baby is still at an increased risk for injury by virtue of being breech.

Nevertheless, most professionals agree that caesarean is the safest option for some breech babies. A number of caregivers, notably Michael Odent, say that in the vast majority of cases they cannot know if a vaginal delivery will be safe until labor has started. They use the first stage of labor as a test. If it goes quickly and all is well, and the mother and baby are both doing fine, then it is a go. However, if the first stage is very long, stops and starts, mother is in a lot of pain or baby is showing signs of distress, they take it as a sign that the baby needs to come into the world by C-section.

What are the chances you actually really need a caesarean? It depends on who you ask. Jane Evans and Mary Cronk, two highly respected UK midwives with significant breech experience, have found that caesareans are necessary in about 20-25% of breech pregnancies. Ina May Gaskin and her colleagues have experienced every kind of breech at their center in Tennessee (99 breech deliveries from 1970-2010). In this (admittedly very small) sample, their total caesarean rate for breech was 10%.

FINDING A CAREGIVER

Your ability to find a local caregiver who attends vaginal breech birth is largely a geographic lottery. In some places, there are a number of midwives who feel confident about breech, and in some places, there is a huge local stigma, fear, or history of litigation concerning breech birth. Remember that vaginal breech birth attended by people who are afraid of breech birth can be very dangerous. Contact people from MyBreechBaby.org or the Coalition for Breech Birth[6] for referrals, or just ask around in your birth community. You may have to travel to have a vaginal breech birth.

---

[6] http://www.aims.org.uk/Journal/Vol10No3/handOffbreech.htm

You can also ask your OB. ACOG explains that if elective caesarean is an option, in spite of its inherent dangers, so must elective vaginal delivery[7] be an option. This does not mean they are going to offer you a vaginal breech birth. It means that your doctor has fiduciary responsibility, so if you want something that is reasonable but she cannot carry it out, she has the duty to support you, find someone who can do it, or figure out a way to make it work. This includes planning a C-section where your baby never leaves you, moving around during labor, and having a vaginal breech birth. Unless there are extenuating circumstances, none of these conditions are unreasonable and you will most likely find someone to support you. You also have the right to tell your doctor she is being unethical when she does not show respect for your decisions, if she uses scare tactics, or if she pressures you into a birth you do not feel good about.

CHANGING BIRTH THROUGH CONSUMER DEMAND

Doctors explain that they do not offer vaginal breech birth because women do not demand vaginal breech birth. At least in the United States, hospitals are businesses. Caesareans bring in more money, and vaginal breech births more risk of litigation. Remember that you are the consumer. You (perhaps through your insurance) are paying for a service. This does not mean you always get what you want, but it means you have the right to full information, to ask, and to be heard. And you also have the right to look elsewhere. If we all take our money, our bodies and our babies away from hospitals that do not offer evidence-based care, they will be forced to change.

Lauren McClain is a childbirth educator who specializes in helping parents of breech babies make decisions about their care. She maintains the website www.mybreechbaby.org. She teaches Birth Boot Camp classes in Maryland and blogs about pregnancy, birth, and parenting at mybreechbaby.org/blog.

■■

---

[7] http://www.mybreechbaby.org/elective-vaginal-delivery.html

Nova McGillivray

Nova had always wanted a natural water birth in the comfort of her own home. After an unplanned caesarean due to a surprise breech, she felt like her world had been torn to shreds. Her feelings of abandonment, isolation, and failure spiraled into depression and anxiety. Many women experience a traumatic birth, but Nova did not let this bring her down – instead, she became actively involved in helping bring about a positive birth culture. She used her birth as a motivator to help other women better prepare and cope with breech babies and caesareans. Her story reminds us that the way a mother feels about her birth experience is extremely important. As painful as it may be to remind yourself about a traumatic birth, you can channel these feelings into something positive.

Surprise Breech, Unplanned Caesarean,
A Reason for Everything

"Never before had I seen such miraculous beauty and yet, I missed the climb."

I took pregnancy and birth quite seriously. Since being a teenager, I thought water birth made perfect sense. My birth would obviously be natural, unmedicated, and without intervention. While trying to conceive, I did some research and found that to have a water birth in my city, it would have to be done at home with midwives. Midwives were at a premium, with there not being enough for every woman who wanted one. I didn't worry – I had faith. Once I learned I was pregnant, I immediately applied to every midwifery clinic in Calgary and surrounding areas. But I never got a midwife, and I accepted that.

I had a 'normal' pregnancy, with the 'usual' minor issues, but I was well prepared. We took a natural childbirth class that included the fathers and encouraged them to play a big role. I chose not to hire a doula – after all, my husband was going to act as my doula. I did the exercises every day throughout the 2nd and 3rd trimesters, I followed the recommended diet, and did all the homework.

At 40 + 3 weeks, I felt all my choices and control slipping away. It turned out the baby was breech. My doctor panicked, and told me I would need surgery that day. I bought a little time, enough to go see my chiropractor and friend for one Webster technique attempt and a good cry in a supportive and safe place.

At the hospital, they offered an ECV (External Cephalic Version), where they tried to manually turn the baby with their hands by pushing on your stomach and the baby inside. I was willing to try anything and everything! Two separate OBs tried. I took deep breaths, closed my eyes and envisioned the baby turning - anything to avoid a C-section. After no success, the attending doctor recommended a C-section as they explained that a vaginal birth was unlikely to be pleasant and possibly unsuccessful anyway. In addition, there were very few doctors that even knew how to deliver a breech baby.

My postpartum depression began shortly after the arrival of my baby. I felt no surprise, excitement, or emotion. My husband was sent home the first three nights, and I was left alone, with the lights on all night and a baby beside my bed, whom I couldn't even pick up by myself. I was not to have her with me in my bed as I might fall asleep and accidentally smother her. I felt lonely, abandoned, isolated, and disconnected from everything due to the drugs. I felt trapped in a small room and physically confined to a bed, unable to roll over or sit up. That started me on a road of anxiety, postpartum depression, breastfeeding and bonding issues, as well as post-traumatic stress disorder symptoms.

Through a lot of effort and work, I have taken many steps to try to appropriately deal with my traumatic birth experience. In fact, that event is what has brought me to finding my passion in my 30's. I am a self-described birth geek. I love making connections with other moms who are active in the positive birth movement and I will read anything birth-related. I wish I could say I am all the way through to the other side, but I still struggle. The simple truth is that I did the best I knew how to at the time, and there should be no guilt and no shame in that.

I like to use my mountain-climbing analogy to reference my birth experience. I trained, I trained hard, I felt completely and totally prepared to climb that mountain and as the date was approaching, I was getting really excited. I showed up at the base of the mountain to check things out as a part of my prep and I was hoisted up in a helicopter. It flew me all the way to the top and dropped me at the summit. I was standing there in awe. Never before had I seen such miraculous beauty and yet, I missed the climb. I never got to experience the triumph and the thrill and the endorphins of climbing that mountain. It is said that you don't always get the birth you want, but you always get the birth you need, and I have made peace with that.

It is said that you don't always get the birth you want, but you always get the birth you need, and I have made peace with that.

If I hadn't have had this experience, I would have never founded ICAN (the International Caesarean Awareness Network), I wouldn't have known there was such a demand for a chapter in my city, and I wouldn't have taken it upon myself to start one. In Alberta, there are chapters in Calgary, Edmonton and Red Deer. If you are recovering from a C-section, want to learn how to avoid one in the first place or are planning a VBAC (Vaginal Birth After Caesarean), I urge you to find us on Facebook or the ICAN website (www.ican-online.org), and attend the meetings. The support and education is so important and inspiring. The

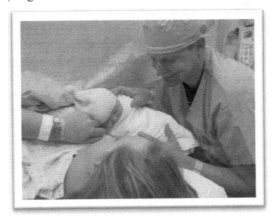

women I have met through ICAN are strong, courageous, and amazing. Just like me. Just like you.

What did you like most about your childbirth experience?

Having my husband there throughout the pregnancy, and during our childbirth classes.

What did you like least about your childbirth experience?

Not being given ALL of my options.

What would you tell an expectant mother to better prepare her for childbirth?

Some of the things I wish I would have known about breech birth, is that first and foremost breech is not an emergency situation! In fact, there are many birthing professionals who say breech presentation is just another variation of normal, so feel free to take your time in making a decision on how you would like to birth. Since it is not an emergency, it is perfectly reasonable to wait to go into labor spontaneously. Even if you plan on having a C-section, your surgery does not need to be scheduled in advance. Even if you are past 40 weeks, the Society of Obstetricians and Gynecologists (SOGC) states that a pregnant woman is not considered overdue until 42 weeks. We do not have accurate ways of estimating the size of the baby, even with ultrasound, so it's simply a guess.

There are OBs who know how to deliver breech, and who are teaching other OBs to do the same. They may not be the norm but they are out there. Don't let anybody tell you it can't be done or "it just isn't done these days," because it can and is being done.

They may not be the norm but they are out there.

Since my birth, I have found a number of doctors in my city who are trained and are actively delivering breech babies with great success. At this time, in Alberta, midwives are not permitted to deliver breech (however in Ontario they are, and I hope Alberta soon follows suit). The midwives know who assists with breech births, and can introduce you to the birth attendants who do. They will sign over your care and as soon as the baby is delivered, the midwives can take you back on as a patient.

Additionally, I would encourage all pregnant women to do up a surgical birth plan, and to look up gentle caesarean, also known as family-centered or mother-centered caesarean. Don't be like me and skip the C-section chapter of the book. Do your research, know your rights. A C-section does not have to be a traumatic experience, as long as you feel like you have been given choices and presented with all options. Have a supportive team of people, and play a role in YOUR birth. Also, hire a doula. I love doulas and would not give birth (vaginally or C-section) again without one.

Finally, remember that you have the RIGHT to decline any intervention.

Finally, remember that you have the RIGHT to decline any intervention.

■■

Webster Technique and Turning a Breech Baby

By Lauren McClain

As I previously mentioned, having a breech baby throws you into a decision-making circus. Do you try to turn the baby? How do you give birth? Should you try an external cephalic version for breech (ECV)? Which of the myriad methods for turning will you pursue? How much time should you spend trying to turn the baby? How much money? When do you stop trying? For when should you schedule a planned caesarean? How far are you willing to travel for a vaginal birth attended by a skilled caregiver?

If you are confident about your birth situation, you may not even want to try to turn the baby. However, for most women, in most places, birth options are greatly decreased with a breech baby. Getting the baby head down relieves a lot of anxiety.

If your baby turns spontaneously (without you doing anything to encourage it), all the better. This does happen, but the likelihood of it happening decreases with every week that passes. If you are 32 weeks or later, and your baby is still breech, it is a good idea to start looking into your options. Keep in mind, though, that at 35 weeks, there is still a 45% chance of your baby turning on its own. At 37 weeks, that drops to 12%. Between 32-36 weeks is generally seen as the most successful window for turning a breech baby.

> *Between 32-36 weeks is generally seen as the most successful window for turning a breech baby.*

These following techniques are all risk-free, and many of them are cost-free as well. One of the most successful ways of turning a breech baby is through chiropractic care. Ideally this care would have started earlier in pregnancy and possibly prevented the breech positioning. A good chiropractor can look at the alignment of your legs and hips early in pregnancy and tell if you are at risk for a breech baby.

The Webster technique (founded by Dr. Larry Webster) can help your body align symmetrically to give the baby the room it needs to feel comfortable moving head-down. It is painless and fast and you can have it done multiple times. Many chiropractors claim high success rates, up to 80%.

How does it work? Imagine your uterus is a latex balloon. The muscles that support and hold it to your body are like strings. If one of them is super tight, it changes the shape of your womb and causes your baby to lay differently. If your uterus or pelvic area is torqued or otherwise stressed or tight, chiropractic care, and especially the Webster technique, is supposed to free baby up to move head down.

If the reason for your baby's breech position is structural (dependent on your body mechanics), positioning exercises and postural changes may also allow baby to turn. In general, use better posture and spend time on your hands and knees. Try these tenets of optimal fetal positioning:

1. When sitting, sit on your butt bones, not on your tail bone, shoulder blades back. Think of the way all the women in Jane Austen movies sit.

2. Always sit with your hips above your knees. Sitting on an exercise ball is great. Couches and recliners are not.

3. Spend at least a few minutes, 3x a day, on hands and knees or in the knee-chest position.

Another way women have found success turning their babies is through hypnosis, relaxation, and/or visualization. A lot has been said on the topic of breech babies born to mothers with high stress levels. We say the baby is trying to stay closer to its mama's heart. An experienced mama-baby hypnotherapist can help, as can listening to relaxation or turning scripts, visualizing your head-down

Another way women have found success turning their babies is through hypnosis, relaxation, and/or visualization.

baby, and generally halting the freak-out train. Relax your mind, relax your body.

Moxibustion and acupuncture have also been used to stimulate a baby to turn in preparation for birth. You can do acupressure yourself or go to an experienced acupuncturist for a more intense session. These techniques correct the energy flow in your body and therefore help your baby align. Moxibustion is sometimes done in complement to acupuncture but often done alone. You can get moxa sticks online or at some health stores. Some practitioners have up to 80% success rate turning babies before 38 weeks.

There is also a host of other simple things people try. The majority of these probably work on babies who will eventually turn anyway, but it is a relief to have the baby turn as soon as possible. Here are some ideas:

> *It is OK. It's perfectly all right to come out feet or butt first.*

1. Put a cold pack on top of the belly and a warm one down low.

2. Shine a light and play music, or have your partner talk to the baby down low.

3. Use peppermint essential oil on top of the belly or myrrh all over.

4. Try belly dancing or rebozo work to loosen the pelvic area.

The irony is that while you work like crazy (or not) to get your baby to turn, the best thing you can do is relax. Get your mind to the place where you are OK with having a breech baby if that's how this baby needs to be born. Tell your baby "It's OK." It is OK. It's perfectly all right to come out feet or butt first.

Lauren McClain is a childbirth educator who specializes in helping parents of breech babies make decisions about their care. She maintains the website www.mybreechbaby.org. She teaches Birth Boot Camp classes in Maryland and blogs about pregnancy, birth, and parenting at mybreechbaby.org/blog.

Lisa Snell

Pregnancy and childbirth can make women feel helpless and hopeless. However, Lisa shares with us the power of faith. When things were not going according to plan, and when obstacle after obstacle kept hindering all efforts, Lisa searched deep within and located her faith. She trusted in God, and understood He had everything under control. She felt happy, under the protection of God, and thus knew her baby would be born in a healthy and positive manner. She knew that everything would be all right.

The Birth of Talia

"There was never a spirit of fear during the whole labor, only peace, even during the most difficult work of my life."

We found out that we were pregnant with our third child on November 8th, which was Philip's 31st birthday. We were quite surprised at God's timing, especially since He began creating a new life in my womb about six months earlier than our 'plan'! Our original due date was July 12th, but after a sonogram, it was established as June 23rd.

At my 34 week appointment, Sharon informed us that baby was still breech. I was surprised at this. I tried not to get concerned, especially when Sharon told me that they like to see baby turned head down by 36 weeks. I figured that I had two weeks and the baby would soon turn. I did begin to go to a chiropractor for the Webster Technique, hoping for a turn. We tried the "breech tilt," and even acupuncture, to no avail.

At 37 weeks, baby was still breech. Now I was beginning to get concerned about my options for the baby's arrival. I had been informed that breech babies were automatically delivered by C-section in Wichita. After having two positive, natural births with our first two children, the thought of a C-section and not a natural birth was a troubling thought.

I scheduled a consultation with Dr. Morgan to talk about the option of an External Version, with a 30% chance of success.

While this didn't seem like good odds to us, we decided that we would go ahead and schedule the version. After all, it was much more preferable than a C-section. I knew that babies could be born breech! The doctor wanted to schedule it for the following Saturday morning. After talking it over with Philip, we decided to turn down that option to honor the Sabbath. The next available time in the schedule was the following Friday, a whole week later.

We made a call to another midwife, Kathy, who we liked immediately. She felt that I was a good candidate for a vaginal delivery of a breech baby and was perfectly willing to assist with the delivery, as long as the baby came before she left town on the 20th.

That night, as I was in bed, I cried as a result of being so frustrated and feeling so out of control. We had been praying that God would turn the baby, yet baby stayed head up. Could I trust God to be glorified in this child's arrival? Would I still be willing to praise God if I had a C-section? These were hard questions for me to answer.

During the last couple weeks of pregnancy, God really used the situation to stretch and grow my faith. At one point, I felt God ask a question: "Who planned this child?" In my frustration, I replied "NOT ME!" He responded, "If I planned this child, do you think that I'd forget to plan the details of its birth?" I knew then God had not forgotten us. He had a plan and I needed to be willing to submit myself to His plan.

He had a plan and I needed to be willing to submit myself to His plan.

On Saturday, June 8th, I was so blessed at the Synagogue to have a group of ladies pray over me. This strengthened and encouraged me.

That night, I was up for about four hours with labor contractions. But after about four hours, the contractions faded and I slept. The next day, I had some sporadic contractions, but nothing seemed too serious. We packed the bags, set up the bassinet, and prepared the overnight bags for the two older kids just in case.

Monday was a normal day. No labor contractions. I was slightly disappointed that labor seemed to have knocked on the door and then left. I woke up at 11:15 pm when my water broke. We were ready, and very calmly, I told Philip what was going on. My first labor contraction came a little after midnight. Contractions were irregularly timed and not very hard. I got out of bed to walk with the contractions.

We got to the Birth Inn at 4:15 am. Kathy met us there, and explained I was 7-8 cm dilated. I was so surprised to be that far along with little to no difficulties. I asked to get into the tub to relax, and that is where I "labored" for the next 45 minutes, listening to some Sue Samuel worship music. Then, around 5:00 am, I had one long and very strong contraction that I was able to relax through with much concentration. At the end of that contraction I was vomiting. When the next contraction came, I was feeling pushy already!

For the next hour and a half I tried my best not to push. This was very difficult and painful, yet God helped. I found that I was best able to suppress the urge to bear down when I had direct eye contact with Kathy and breathed with her. Baby had a strong heart rate the whole time and was slowly moving down with each contraction. Finally, after an hour and a half of breathing through pushing contractions, I simply could not not push. I was clear to push without running any risk of injuring my sweet baby. With a couple contractions, I pushed baby's feet and bottom out at the same time. That was big. And then, the

contraction faded and I desperately waited for the next contraction to push against. With that one, baby came out to the chest. This was the most exciting part of birthing

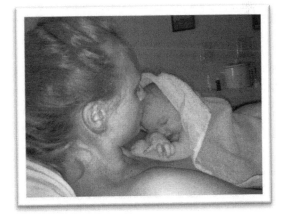

our baby! Baby wasn't even born yet, but we exclaimed, "IT'S A GIRL!" We were able to call our baby girl out by name. Talia Joy! Come on, girl! She got her arms down, turned her head just the right way, and Kathy caught her on the way down.

Up on my chest, she cried briefly, and was nursing within ten minutes. Healthy, beautiful, 7lbs, 10oz, and dark hair. A natural breech birth. To God be the glory! There was never a spirit of fear during the whole labor, only peace, even during the most difficult work of my life.

What did you like most about your childbirth experience?

My favorite part of this birth story is the faithfulness in God! He really saw us through a scary time of uncertainty and gave my husband and me peace, instead of fear. This is a life lesson that was taught to us throughout this birthing process.

What did you like least about your childbirth experience?

What I didn't like about this birthing process is mostly all the politics and policies that were brought into light in the hospital setting. I very much disliked being told that I would have a C-section just because my baby was breech.

What would you tell an expectant mother to better prepare her for childbirth?

On every level, prepare for birth and prepare to become a mother. It is easy to get so knowledgeable about the birthing process and forget that God has something incredible to teach you spiritually, emotionally, and relationally with your spouse during pregnancy, labor, birth, and motherhood. Enter into it with an attitude of prayer! Also, surround yourself with positive birth stories. Nothing is more discouraging than hearing endless horror stories about labor and people praising the "simplicity" of C-sections.

In Transition

Despite hospital and home births being the two usual birthing environment options that women are presented with, some women actually give birth somewhere in between. The following two stories will certainly give you an adrenaline rush, but are also meant to show you that birth might occur on its own terms. The baby will decide when it is ready to be born. To stop the birth would mean to intervene, and to intervene would mean to throw labor off its natural course. It is OK to let labor unfold on its own. It is OK to allow our bodies to birth babies without (unnecessary) intervention.

Phyllis Roberts

An experience does not beget that same experience. You are not subject to repeat the same feelings. Unlike for her first two, Phyllis found the strength to take more control over her third childbirth, and decided to have it without medication and as natural as possible. She wanted to decide in what manner she would give birth. In the end, she and her husband delivered her baby in an unexpected location. Her story does not intend to scare women, but rather depicts her courage, faith, and excellent preparation for childbirth. She knew exactly what to do and how to do it because she understood how childbirth works, and more importantly, she believed in herself. She let nature help guide her, and surrendered herself to the magic.

The Birth of My Baby

"It was like all the strength that I possessed went to that one spot, to birth my little girl."

My name is Phyllis. I am 27 years old, and my daughter was born in the parking lot of Bay Area Midwifery Center in Annapolis, Maryland.

My first two childbirth experiences were OK. I had an epidural with both. I was pretty much talked into them by my OB/GYN. At the time, I didn't know that any other way to give birth even existed. Especially not for average young moms like myself. Seven years later, my husband and I were pregnant again. After more than one miscarriage, we were ecstatic.

This time around, I planned on being more educated and involved in determining how I would give birth. Most of all, I was outraged at how little faith society, and especially medical professionals, had in a woman's body. I didn't understand why they expected us to be unable to give birth without intervention. Why did they expect us to need medicine? Why did they downplay the importance of having your childbirth the way you wanted to?

I was much more educated on a woman's right to have a fair chance at her ideal birth experience. I planned to have a natural, vaginal birth, in a dimly lit room or birthing tub. I enlisted the help of a doula, for free. I found a birth center that was an hour away from my home and I decided to have my prenatal care handled by a nurse midwife. I noticed the difference at once. My midwife trusted my body and was very personable. My doula was empowering, reassuring, very resourceful, open and honest. I felt amazing, awesome, and so strong.

My EDD was April 1st, but my midwife assured me that my baby would arrive when she was ready, and that EDDs are just that – Estimated Due Dates. On April 4th at around 5 pm, I started contracting every 5-7 minutes. Contractions were very strong, but I was handling them like a champ. I think this may have caused me to underestimate how REAL my labor was.

Contractions were very strong, but I was handling them like a champ.

That night, I continued walking through the house, contracting, breathing, squatting, and such. My husband timed my contractions, and sure enough they were every 5-6 minutes, lasting a little more than one minute. I remember feeling so capable and confident that I could do this. My doula had provided me with very effective breathing techniques, and I had read a few books that offered helpful advice. I labored all night with regular contractions.

At about 4 am, my husband and I began to get ready. I took a shower, which helped tremendously. We arrived at the birthing center and my midwife checked me. She said I was 1 cm dilated. I was very upset because those contractions felt like I would be at least 4 cm along!

We decided to go to my mom's house because she lived closer to the center. As we were driving, I was still experiencing contractions. I noticed that watching the clock helped and encouraged me because it put everything into perspective. This one minute of work (pain) would bring me closer to seeing my new baby. I became excited.

I now realize that I began the transition into 'labor land' at my mom's. I became unresponsive as family tried to talk to me. I wanted to be left alone in peace and quiet. I got down on all fours on her floor, and continued to breathe while repeating my affirmation.

I got down on all fours again, this time on the bathroom floor. My husband came in to check on me, as I had been gone for several minutes. He looked at me and immediately knew we should leave. I tried to reassure him that it would be several more hours like this. Just then, my water broke. My husband called my midwife and told her we were heading to the center. During the trip back, I was repeating my affirmation while contracting. When we arrived in the birth center parking lot, I was grunting and bearing down in the passenger seat of our car. I had an overwhelming urge to push, so I did. Once my husband parked, he came over to open my door. I let out a scream, got up, and tried walking. I didn't even make it 3 feet before I had another urge to push. So I did. With that push my daughter's head began to crown. I grabbed his hand and allowed him to feel. His mouth fell open.

I then had another urge to push, and began to drop to my knees. My husband pulled me up. I took a few steps, and then wanted to push again. My husband quickly dialed our midwife to tell her I could no longer move. I got down on all fours. Another push, and her shoulders came out. My husband got down under me, and then I knew this was it. I let out a scream and a push. The burning sensation, although painful, was amazing and powerful. It was like all the strength that I possessed went to that one spot, to birth my

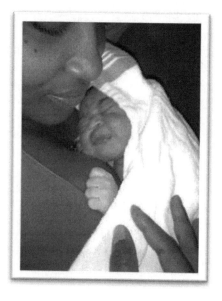

little girl. With that final big push, she emerged. My husband caught her and held her close to his body. My midwife ran up the stairs and yelled, looking for us. We laughed and told her where we were. A priest also came over to see if we were OK.

I sat in a wheelchair, holding my daughter. The umbilical cord was still attached as the priest, my husband, and my midwife rolled me into the birthing center. Ten minutes later, my doula showed up asking if she could at least get me a drink. It was the most beautiful thing to ever happen to me. If I could go back in time and change it, I wouldn't. I would keep it exactly the way it was. It was perfect!

What did you like most about your childbirth experience?

I liked how unexpected it was and how much I surprised myself by being so strong.

What did you like least about your childbirth experience?

Honestly, my only dislike is the fact that it happened so fast. We were unable to take pictures.

What would you tell an expectant mother to better prepare her for childbirth?

I would tell all expectant mothers to consider all scenarios when planning their birth. Women should know that things may stray away from the plan, but that does not make it any less of a great experience. I would suggest a lot of positive self-affirmations every day. And a doula. Doulas, along with positive self-affirmations, made me feel extremely capable of giving birth (naturally). For my first two

Doulas, along with positive self-affirmations, made me feel extremely capable of giving birth (naturally).

pregnancies, I had convinced myself I couldn't do it. These positive thoughts and affirmations, along with the support from my doula, really made me feel confident that I could do this.

For those who may find themselves in an unexpected location:

In my opinion, the best reaction would be to remain calm and focused. Truthfully, I think we don't give our bodies enough credit. Once I came to the realization that she was coming, all I could think about was birthing my baby. I did not notice much of anything else going on around me in the parking lot. I was all at once very hypersensitive, while drowning out almost all of my surroundings.

Your best reaction would be joy; joy that you are going to meet your little one. My husband and I were so excited we kept telling each other "I can't believe this, it's so awesome." Do not overthink your birth and do not stress out about it. It's great to plan and prepare, but the truth **is,** female bodies have been doing this forever! I trusted my body in that parking lot. Your body knows what to do, so go with the flow and rejoice!

Your body knows what to do, so go with the flow and rejoice!

Lea Lion

If you've been following birth stories for a while, you may have heard of our next story. Lea gave birth in a hospital parking lot. Despite not expecting this scenario, she and her husband reacted perfectly during this surreal experience. They did not panic, but let the birth unfold naturally and peacefully. They did not fear it, but rather cooperated beautifully and brought their baby into this world in a normal and natural fashion. Her story encourages all women to not wait frantically for birth to come, but to let it happen at its own pace, when it is time.

The Birth of My Baby

"Your body is designed to do it! You are strong. You can do it! Just don't forget to breathe."

Having a baby in a parking lot is not what I thought I would become known for, but it was one of the best experiences of my life and, luckily, I love telling -- and retelling -- my birth story.

A watched pot never boils. At three days past my due date with my second child, I knew what it felt like to be the pot. Every time I came downstairs -- in the morning, after a midday nap, before dinner -- my in-laws, who were in town for the birth, observed, "Still no baby?"

I tried walking and yoga and sex to bring on labor. There was nothing left to do except ride mini-trains, my then 2-year-old's latest obsession. As I squeezed myself in behind the steering wheel to drive home, I felt a cramp coming on like a gentle wave. I didn't tell anybody. I knew if I told my parents, the watched pot phenomenon would intensify and, besides, I knew from my first birth that I still had a long journey ahead of me.

At home, my husband and I watched a movie -- no idea which one though -- I was too busy concentrating on the wave-like sensation that rolled through my belly every half hour. "The babe is on the way," I told my husband.

At 2:00 am, I was up again, so I read a few birth stories from "Spiritual Midwifery" by Ina May Gaskin, to get in the baby-having mood. The waves were stronger now -- coming about every 20 minutes -- but still far from the all-encompassing contractions that I remembered.

When I felt a contraction coming on, I would leap out of bed and start circling our Oriental rug only to have the wave fade away without ever reaching the crescendo of my memory.

At sunrise, after hours of mellow waves, I had two body-rocking contractions in a row. The intensity of giving birth came rushing back to me. I remembered, in the middle of active labor, thinking about how easy running a marathon must be in comparison. I got into my favorite birthing position -- standing with my arms wrapped around my husband's neck -- and moaned.

A contraction crashed through me. I could feel the baby's head crown and then, as the contraction subsided, it got sucked back into the birth canal. "We have to go!" I yelled.

There was no way I could sit down. Every time I had a contraction, the baby's head would emerge a little bit more. So I kneeled backwards in the passenger seat and held onto the leather headrest. I moaned. My husband called our obstetrician on speakerphone. We pulled into the hospital parking lot, and my husband jumped out. He opened my door and started getting our bags out of the trunk.

Standing at last, I had another contraction. I reached my hand down and felt the top of the baby's head. "I'm having the baby right now," I said.

My husband dropped down onto his knees. He dropped the car keys. He didn't have time to drop the bags that were slung over his chest. I stood with my hands on my thighs. My husband was behind me. One more push and the baby's head popped out. Then my water broke and a huge splash of fluid drenched my husband, the baby and the parking lot floor. I felt the

One more push and the baby's head popped out.

baby's body slide out -- fast, really fast -- into my husband's open hands.

When the baby was out, I tried to take a step forward, but the umbilical cord yanked me back into place. Immediately, the baby started to cry. When we heard his cries, a wave of relief washed over us. "Hi baby," "Oh my God," "Hi baby," we chanted again and again. It was cold and damp and I gathered the long skirt of my dress to wrap around him. My husband hugged him close.

The parking lot -- one of the busiest in L.A. -- was deserted. Minutes passed. Eventually, I saw a parking lot attendant in the distance. "We just had a baby!" I yelled.

"We just had a baby!" I yelled.

More minutes passed. Then, the elevator doors opened and three nurses came running out into the parking lot, each pushing a wheelchair.

It was pandemonium. Nurses shouting. Wheelchairs flying. Baby crying. What was going on? Why were there so many wheelchairs?

"Pass the baby to me," one of the nurses instructed my husband. She held out her arms, urging him to hand the baby through my legs.

"I'm not passing my baby anywhere," he replied. "Are you crazy?"

Before she had a chance to answer, our doctor arrived, took charge and started yelling at the nurses. "Where are my clamps? Where are blankets? Why are there so many wheelchairs?"

My husband remained behind me, holding the baby, and the baby and I were still attached by the umbilical cord. There was only one thing to do.

"Lea, do you think you could swing your leg over my head and turn around?" my husband asked.

After giving birth? No problem. I did a fan kick over my husband's head and with the cord now in front of me, sat down in one of the wheelchairs. My husband handed the baby to me and I got my first full on look at my new baby boy.

We went up to the maternity floor in a blissful, post-birth bubble. But once we got there, it was chaos again.

Dozens of doctors and nurses and hospital administrators squeezed into our delivery room. I delivered the placenta in one easy push. I breastfed my new baby. The nurses took the baby over to the scale and weighed him. It was business as usual -- except that no one seemed to be able to figure out how to check us -- a mother and a baby -- into the maternity ward.

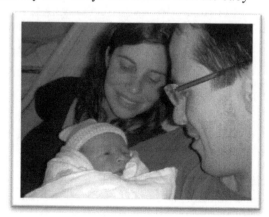

What did you like most about your childbirth experience?

My birth experience was divine. My body and my baby did everything exactly as they were designed to do, and my baby boy was born – in the amniotic sac! – and into his father's open arms. It was powerful! We got to welcome him into the world together and spend the first moments of his life just the three of us. It goes to show that moments of pure joy can happen anywhere – even in a parking lot. And, of course, I love a good birth story.

What did you like least about your childbirth experience?

Dealing with the hospital bureaucracy. Apparently, there is no official form to check a mother and a baby into the hospital. That took a while to sort out. Also, someone from the billing department immediately began harassing us about our health insurance information (we had it). We also had just had a baby minutes before! I was breastfeeding. We weren't going anywhere. It seemed like the insurance situation could wait.

Then, a couple weeks after the birth, we received an exorbitantly overcharged bill from the hospital that included fees for anesthesia (I didn't have it, obviously) and a labor room (didn't use that one either!)

Did you consider giving birth at home once you realized the baby was coming?

In retrospect, I should have just stayed at home to have the baby. I could have avoided the car ride, the parking lot and the hospital bureaucracy. It would certainly have been more comfortable and probably cleaner. In the moment (and in active labor!) the thought didn't cross my mind. We had such a positive experience with natural childbirth in a hospital with our first son, so we just wanted to do it again. Of course, as every parent knows, every child (and every birth) is completely different and new. Our second birth was much, much faster. I can say with no doubt that if I ever have another baby, I will plan a home birth!

What would you tell an expectant mother to better prepare her for childbirth?

Be as healthy as possible in your mind and your body. Eat nutritious food, green vegetables and fresh fruit, get loads of exercise, go outside, do yoga, meditate. Birth is very physical but it is also mental. Visualize your birth, think about the details, create a positive birth environment, find a guide (partner, midwife, doctor) who supports you and makes you feel empowered. Read "Spiritual Midwifery" by Ina May Gaskin and have your partner read it too. Go with the flow no matter what happens.

Here are some of the things I asked my husband to remind me of during labor: Women have been having babies for thousands of years, your grandmother did it, your mother did it, your body is designed to do it! You are strong. You can do it! Just don't forget to breathe.

Home Births

Our third and final segment in this book features a series of home births. A hospital birth has become such a norm in many countries, that the very thought of having a home birth is quite controversial. However, for low-risk pregnancies, home birth is often a viable option. Birth support may include highly-qualified midwives, doulas, or just family members. Women who have given birth at home have expressed an overwhelming degree of joy and pure bliss. Others have also mentioned that even though there may have been a few unexpected circumstances, they nevertheless felt magnificent. While a home birth may not be desired by all, or even attainable, many women found that the familiarity of their own home and surroundings actually facilitated their birth. It made the experience truly personal. Please enjoy the following stories, as they really are full of peace, tranquility, and happiness.

■■■

Tiffany Jerry

Tiffany shares with us her two birth stories. Both took place under the kind help of a midwife, but the first occurred in a hospital, and the second in Tiffany's home. This transition to a home birth from a hospital one can also be seen at the macro-level, with more and more women finding that they will feel more comfortable and happy birthing at home. Tiffany explains the power it took to birth her babies, but also the sense of triumph that she felt knowing that she had birthed naturally and as she had wanted.

The Births of My Two Babies

"It was like climbing the highest mountain with an elephant on my back, but it made me even more proud in the end."

I am 21 years old. I have just walked home from a stressful day at work. As I sit on the couch, still 9 days away from my 'due date,' I realize my stomach is hurting. It comes and goes, on and off, and I think nothing of it but that perhaps I overdid it with my 45 minute walk home.

At 2 am, I am awoken by cramps that won't let me sleep. I watch some silly movie and ride it out. I fall asleep on the couch when the cramps dissipate around 7 am. My boyfriend goes to work, and the cramps stay away all day. He arrives home again at 9 pm to see that my cramps are back. We wonder if it's labor, but are quite sceptical. We decide to go for a walk to get some ice cream. On the walk, the cramping gets stronger, and more regular, happening every 10-12 minutes, making me stop walking. We get home and rest for the evening, timing the contractions, at 10 minutes, then 8 minutes, then 4 minutes apart by 5 am. At 5:30 am, we start calling our midwives, to find they are either sleeping off previous births or attending to new ones. A midwife from another team arrives at our one-bedroom basement apartment by 7 am.

I am 4 cm dilated. We decide to head to the hospital, 45 minutes away. It's the worst ride of my life. I vomit and try to sleep between contractions. We arrive at the hospital at 7:45 am. I am not hooked up to anything. My midwife suggests I jump in the shower for some relief. I am now 8 cm dilated. I spend what seems like an eternity in the shower (but reality tells me it was about 30 minutes), loving the sweet relief it gives, before the overwhelming urge to push kicks in. I get back to the bed, and 12 minutes later my beautiful 6lbs 8oz daughter is born healthy, crying, and I am blessed. We arrive home 6 hours later and are greeted by family.

12 minutes later my beautiful 6lbs 8oz daughter is born healthy, crying, and I am blessed.

I am 25 years old. I am getting married in 3 days to the father of my first child, the love of my life. I have just taken a test and found out that I am pregnant. We are overjoyed, though shocked it happened so fast! We just started trying this month. The pregnancy is smooth, despite severe morning sickness and some non-threatening bleeding.

We have a dinner party with some friends; I am 37+6 weeks pregnant. I am awakened to pressure and wetness at 3:45 am. In a daze, I get out of bed, change my PJ pants, and discover the wetness isn't stopping. With slow realization, I come to understand that my water has broken. I return to bed, thinking I have some time to waste. I time contractions every 5-8 minutes for an hour. I am feeling nauseous.

At 5:20 am, I wake my husband to tell him the news. He blows up the tub downstairs, and we leave our 4 year old daughter to sleep. At 5:40 am, we call the midwives. Again, just my luck, my first midwife is attending a birth. The others are not on call, but one of them comes anyways. She arrives at 6:20 am and is wonderful.

I am 3-4 cm dilated. I am sipping water and folding laundry in our small three-bedroom home. The contractions make me stand up each time they arrive. In just a few hours, I go from 3-4 cm to fully dilated. Midwife #1, Natalie, arrives and relieves Martha, the midwife who came even though she was not on call. Natalie breaks my 2nd bag of water, as I've been sitting at 10 cm for a long time with no urge to push. No one knew because the contractions, though intense, were not hard to cope through.

Within 15 minutes, at exactly 1:00 pm, my second child is born. I meet my son. Pushing was the most intense feeling I've ever felt. It was like climbing the highest mountain with an elephant on my back, but it made me even more proud in the end. He's a succulent 8lbs 7oz baby. We lay on the couch, soaking in the love for an hour or so, and then I hand him to daddy. He's in love too

Natalie stays for about 2 hours, checking on us, giving us information, and then leaves us to bond, with her pager number right beside me. She got soaked to her under arms when I was in my final stages, so she leaves wearing one of my husband's t-shirts. She'll be back in 24 hours, to return it. We are so happy.

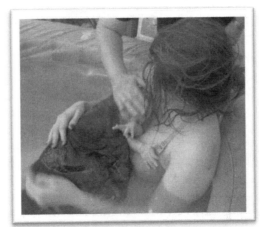

Why the change from hospital to home birth?

When we chose a hospital birth with our first child, there were many uneducated reasons for this decision, but reasons nonetheless. I wanted the experience of "bringing baby home." We lived in a small one-bedroom apartment, and I felt we didn't have enough room. The cleanup involved wasn't appealing, and of course, being my first time, I had no idea what to expect. So, a hospital with all of its options and choices seemed like a smart, safe idea.

Once I knew what childbirth was, knew more about the safety of home birth, and after watching several birthing documentaries, we decided a home birth was for us. Not having to travel during contractions, the comfort of my bed/couch after birth, my own food, not having to find childcare for my oldest, no nurses, no bad hospital smell, no outside germs, the option to birth in a tub, all of these things helped me choose home birth. I cannot imagine now going back to a hospital to deliver any future babies.

What did you like most about your childbirth experience?

The support! I can never imagine giving birth in a situation where a doctor comes and goes, and where different nurses come and go. I want to know who's going to see me and support me in my most vulnerable moments! I want someone who's going to hold me up, encourage me, and see me through it from start to end. The peace of mind my midwife afforded me through her support, as well as her patience, was the best part of my childbirth experience.

What did you like least about your childbirth experience?

Funny enough, my least favorite part is that the perineal massage I was given didn't happen often enough! It's quite embarrassing, however, when the perineal massage was given, my pain was temporarily forgotten, as the sensation of gentleness down there was blissful. It took my mind off the acute pressure. I was too embarrassed to say anything because I felt they would see it as awkward. Midwives

When the perineal massage was given, my pain was temporarily forgotten.

and doctors, take note! It's a wonderful gift to give, those massages!

What would you tell an expectant mother to better prepare her for childbirth?

A mother should know that she is strong. It is of utmost importance that she 100% believes she can do it. Her mindset will be the deciding factor as to whether she gets through her natural birth or not.

She should have a great support network. She needs to know she is going to have people to back her up. She needs to make her needs clear to those people. She needs a strong birth plan. She needs to trust her backup and care providers with 100% certainty.

She should be informed; educated on every aspect of birth. What's healthiest for mom, for baby, etc.? What long term effects do birth practises have on mother and baby? How can dad be of assistance? What's the role of a doula, does she want one? What resources can she use before and after?

I also want her to know that she is not alone, that she is gorgeous and brave and meant for this. That whatever she feels is normal, that billions have done it before her, and that she will be OK.

> *That whatever she feels is normal, that billions have done it before her, and that she will be OK.*

Perineal Protectors

Rachel Reed

Perineal tearing and/or grazing is common during birth. Two thirds of women will sustain damage to their perineum during birth (AIHW 2012). For most, this consists of tearing or grazing, and for around 12% the damage is caused by an episiotomy.

When summarizing a birth, midwives often end with 'and an intact perineum,' to which the reply is usually 'well done'. However, claiming of responsibility for perineal outcome also works in reverse. If a woman sustains an extensive tear, the midwife is blamed and her practice questioned by colleagues and herself. So, is there really anything anyone can do to avoid perineal damage during birth?

According to research, most of the risk factors for perineal tearing are out of the control of the midwife, and to a large extent, out of the control of the mother as well. Influencing factors include[8]:

- A big baby
- High weight gain in pregnancy
- Higher socioeconomic circumstances
- Older and younger maternal age
- Ethnicity (Caucasian and Asian)
- First vaginal birth

The controllable factors that influence perineal damage are:

PREPARATION

For first time mothers, perineal stretching massage during pregnancy can reduce the chance of tearing (Albers et al.

---

[8] (Albers et al. 2006; Dahlen et al. 2007; Goldberg et al. 2003; Groutz et al. 2011; Helain et al. 2011; Lydon-Rochelle et al. 1995; Mayerhofer et al. 2002; Murphy & Feinland 1998; Nodine & Roberts 1987; Shorten et al. 2002; Soong & Barnes 2005)

2005; Beckmann & Garrett 2007). Carolyn Hastie has designed an excellent leaflet explaining exactly how to do this. Perineal stretching massage can increase a woman's confidence in her body's ability to stretch and open for her baby. On the other hand, plenty of women don't prepare in this way and whether you have confidence in your body or not, your perineum will stretch. It is also important for women to know that it is normal for the perineum to tear, and that if it does, they have not 'failed'.

There is a rather scary device called an Epi-No designed to use during pregnancy to stretch the perineum. The limited research regarding the effectiveness and safety of this device is inconclusive (Kovacs, Heath & Campbell 2004; Shek et al. 2011). Personally, I worry about potential long term effects of repeatedly stretching the perineum to the size of a baby's head. Although a woman may give birth a number of times during her life, she will usually have more than a day between each baby's head stretching her vagina. It is also a reflection of our technocratic culture that a 'device' is considered to be necessary in order to prepare for childbirth.

> *It is also a reflection of our technocratic culture that a 'device' is considered to be necessary in order to prepare for childbirth.*

POSITIONS

Lateral and hands-knees positions reduce the chance of tearing, and supine, squatting or lithotomy positions increase the chance of tearing (Albers et al. 1996; Hastings-Tolsma et al. 2007; Mayerhofer et al. 2002; Murphy & Feinland 1998; Shorten, Donsante & Shorten 2002). I have noticed that when women are left to birth instinctively, they will often move from a squatting position – if they got into one – into a hands-knees position just before the head crowns. In forward leaning positions, any tearing that does occur will usually be labial rather than vaginal. Labial tears sting like mad but heal well.

WARM WATER

A warm flannel held against the perineum during crowning can reduce the incidence of major tearing and reduce postnatal pain and urinary incontinence (Dahlen et al. 2007; Hastings-Tolsma et al. 2007). A recent Cochrane Review also supported the use of warm compresses to decrease the occurrence of perineal trauma. However, for some women this is intrusive and irritating. Water birth is fabulous for avoiding tears – and makes it difficult for anyone apart from the birthing woman to touch the perineum or baby during birth.

PERINEAL MASSAGING DURING BIRTH

Massaging the perineum as the baby is trying to be born concerns me for a number of reasons. It makes me really uncomfortable to watch a lot of 'activity' being done to a woman's body while she is trying to birth. I have seen some very brutal versions of 'perineal massage' done to women. However, the Cochrane Review suggests that this type of massaging can reduce the chance of significant tears (3rd and 4th degree), although this does not make it into their conclusion. These types of tearing are rare (around 1%), so the intervention needs to be weighed up with the risk.

SLOW BIRTH OF THE BABY'S HEAD

A slow birth of the baby's head reduces the chance of tearing. It allows the tissues to gently stretch over time as the baby moves forward with each contraction and retracts afterwards – two steps forward and one step back. A study by Albers et al. (2006) concluded that birthing the baby's head between contractions slows the birth down and 'requires a joint effort by the mother and her clinician'. Yet another example of how misguided research can be, and a reflection of how inherent our mistrust of women's bodies is. I can only find one study that has bothered to look at what women do when we leave them alone. This extremely small study of 4 women birthing without instructions (imagine that!) found that they altered their own

breathing and stopped pushing as the baby's head crowned
(Aderhold & Robert's 1991). It's a shame research into
physiological birth is so limited. Instead I will have to rely on
experiential knowledge…

INSTINCTIVE MATERNAL BEHAVIOR VS. INSTRUCTION

Coached pushing increases the chance of perineal
tearing, and this may be because it interferes with the instinctive
response during crowning. The intense sensations experienced
during crowning usually result in the woman 'holding back'
while the uterus continues to push the baby out slowly and
gently. Often women will hold their baby's head and/or their
vulva. I have witnessed one mother attempt to push her baby
back in. It was unsuccessful, but gave us a giggle afterwards.
Telling a woman to stop pushing, pant or 'give little pushes'
distracts her at a crucial moment and suggests that she is not the
expert in her birth. She is the one with a baby's head in her
vagina – leave it to her.

Some women will close their legs during crowing. I have
seen midwives push women's legs back open or say 'keep your
legs open'. Closing the legs, or bringing them in from a wide-
open position protects the perineum.
The two positions that involve the least
chance of tearing (left lateral and
hands/knees) do not involve stretched
out legs and therefore perineums. As for
whether closing your legs will stop a
baby from coming out… it may slow it
down, but that baby is coming out. I
have seen a woman birth on her side
with her legs crossed – her baby came
out from behind.

I have seen a woman birth on her side with her legs crossed – her baby came out from behind.

'HANDS ON' TECHNIQUES

Hands on techniques aimed at slowing the birth of the
baby and supporting the perineal tissues are routinely used by
many birth attendants. In summary, research findings explain

'hands on' approaches may or may not reduce the chance of minor tearing, but increase the chance of episiotomy and major tearing (Mayerhofer et al. 2002 McCandlish et al. 1998). No research has compared instinctive physiological birth (no epidurals, induction etc.) with a 'hands on' approach. In addition, no research has explored women's experiences of a 'hands on' approach. Ideally, this should be discussed before labor, and the mother should choose the approach she would like. For some individual women, a 'hands on' approach may be appropriate. For example, some women with previous tearing want the psychological comfort of a 'hands on' approach.

Perineal massage during the birth of the head has been found to reduce the chance of significant tearing i.e. 3rd or 4th degree (Aasheim, et al. 2011). However, in Australia, only 1.7% of women sustain this level of tearing (AIHW 2011) and this technique is very invasive. The use of this technique should be discussed and agreed upon during pregnancy.

Perineal massage during the birth of the head has been found to reduce the chance of significant tearing.

EPISIOTOMY

An episiotomy does not prevent a tear from occurring. Instead, it increases the chance of a 3rd or 4th degree tear (involving the anal sphincter). Even in obstetric guidelines, an episiotomy is not recommended as a way to protect the perineum during birth. Although an episiotomy is easier to suture, a natural tear is less painful and heals quicker. The only excuse for cutting an episiotomy is for an instrumental birth or for a baby who needs to be born quickly.

SUTURING

Suturing is the most common method of perineal repair. Whether to suture or not should be the woman's decision. In relation to 2nd degree tears (the most common), the need to suture is debatable if the tear aligns well and is not bleeding. A recent Cochrane review concluded:

"…at present there is insufficient evidence to suggest that one method is superior to the other with regard to healing and recovery in the early or late postnatal periods. Until further evidence becomes available, clinicians' decisions whether to suture or not can be based on their clinical judgment and the woman's preference after informing them about the lack of long-term outcomes and possible chance of slower wound healing process, but possible better overall feeling of wellbeing if left un-sutured." (Elharmeel et al. 2011)

In my own experience as a midwife, I have found that un-sutured perineums heal very quickly and with far less pain than sutured perineums. Nowadays, my suturing skills are mostly utilized in teaching suturing.

IN SUMMARY

There is very little that midwives can do to protect women's perineums, so they need to stop taking the credit and the blame for perineal outcome. Instead, women need to be encouraged to trust that their body has an innate ability to birth their baby; that perineal tearing is a normal part of birth; and that the body will heal itself.

Women need to be encouraged to trust that their body has an innate ability to birth their baby; that perineal tearing is a normal part of birth; and that the body will heal itself.

Dr. Rachel Reed is a Lecturer at the University of the Sunshine Coast and a home birth midwife. She has practised midwifery in a range of models and settings in the United Kingdom and Australia. Rachel is committed to the promotion of physiological birth, and of women's innate ability to birth and mother. She is a writer and presenter and is also the author of the MidwifeThinking blog site: www.midwifethinking.com.

Rachel Hasell

Whereas some expectant moms worry that their labor may take too long, Rachel took a different approach to birth. She decided to have a VBAC home birth after recognizing that her body delivered babies more quickly than the average woman. There was an attempt to pressure Rachel into birthing in a hospital, but Rachel found the support she needed to give birth at home, in a comfortable and relaxing atmosphere. She had a peaceful and pleasant birth. Her story is a beautiful example of how giving birth can be such a joyous event.

The Birth of Henry

"It was such a beautiful family birth, just perfect."

I had my second baby, Henry, at home. It was such a relaxed and beautiful birth, completely different from the birth of my first baby, Emi, in the hospital. I felt so supported and empowered by my midwives. They really did provide individualized care rather than conveyor belt care. It made such a difference seeing the same couple of midwives throughout my pregnancy, birth and postnatal time. My husband and I were able to build a good relationship with our first on-call midwife. When I went into labor, I felt like I was calling a trusted friend who really knew me, rather than a stranger. In the ideal world, this is just how midwifery care should be for everyone.

My first labor, with our daughter, was very quick and relatively easy, although I ended up with an emergency caesarean section at the pushing stage. I had an undiagnosed breech with unsurprisingly, thick meconium and also fetal distress. My waters went 36 hours before my contractions began, and I ended up with an infection, which meant her heart rate was abnormally high. After discussing a vaginal breech birth, with an open-minded obstetrician on duty, we opted for an emergency caesarean, as we didn't want to stress Emi any more.

I wasn't a typical candidate for choosing a home birth the second time around. As it was such a quick labor the first time, I was anxious about laboring even more quickly the second time, and not making it to the hospital in time.

The midwives at my local hospital were very supportive of my decision. The VBAC specialist consultant also respected my decision, and was refreshingly supportive and normality-focused. I had initially been very disheartened when another consultant at a different hospital had been very patronizing, and strongly disagreed with me having a VBAC at home. It was wonderful to have midwives and a doctor who believed that I could successfully labor and birth at home.

It was wonderful to have midwives and a doctor who believed that I could successfully labor and birth at home.

I went into spontaneous labor with our son Henry at 40+2 weeks on October 20th, 2013. I had a show the day before, and went for a couple of long walks. I then started having very mild, irregular tightenings at about 9:15 pm. It was so lovely and relaxed, my husband Dave and I pottered around the kitchen, listening to jazz music and making banana muffins. When the contractions started to come more regularly, I breathed through them, and used my hypnobirthing techniques, while Dave massaged my back. At about 9:50 pm, the contractions were becoming more regular, and I started having to focus and to breathe through them more, so I called our lovely midwife.

She arrived at 10:30 pm, and quietly set things up and supported me, as Dave started filling the pool. She examined me at 10:45 pm and I was 6 cm dilated. I was so relieved, as I thought she might say 'sorry you're only in early labor'. By this point the contractions were much more intense. I then got in the pool, which was so calming and relaxing. It really helped me 'zone out,' and just let my body get on with it. My sister and mum arrived at 11:15 pm, just in time to look after our 2 year old daughter who woke up. I then started feeling lots of pressure and spontaneously bearing down at 11:30 pm.

Our midwife called the second midwife, who arrived after baby Henry did! This part of my labor was incredibly intense, and a little overwhelming. It felt very animalistic. I'd felt in control up to that point, but then my body just took over.

I put my hand down and felt the top of his head, which was just visible at 11:40 pm, and with one big push he was born at 11:44 pm. I lifted him out of the water, the midwife unwrapped the cord, and we had our lovely first cuddle. Those first few moments together were so precious, and I'll remember them forever. Our daughter Emi came in minutes after he was born, and laughed with delight at the "tiny, cute baby in the swimming pool." Emi started taking her pyjamas off and trying to get in the pool for a cuddle with the tiny baby! It was such a beautiful family birth, just perfect. I'm so glad I didn't have to drive to the hospital, worrying whether we'd make it in time. It was so relaxed, just like an episode of "Call the Midwife."

I had a physiological placental delivery, with minimal blood loss and some suturing for a 2nd degree tear. It was such an amazing feeling knowing that I did it! The midwives cleaned everything up, (there really was no mess left when I got up the following morning!) and tucked us all up in bed. Perfect.

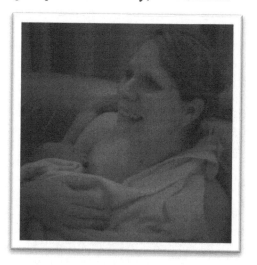

What did you like most about your childbirth experience?

I felt so relaxed and empowered. A truly life-affirming and beautiful experience. It was wonderful to have a shower in my own bathroom afterwards, then sit in an armchair breastfeeding, and have tea and toast while the midwives did their paperwork.

Afterwards, it was so blissful to sleep in my own bed, snuggled up with my husband and baby just hours after giving birth. I loved that it was a family experience in our own home, rather than being clinical and rushed.

> *I loved that it was a family experience in our own home, rather than being clinical and rushed.*

What did you like least about your childbirth experience?

One consultant at another hospital strongly disagreed with our decision to have a VBAC at home. I initially felt guilty, humiliated and powerless.

I was so glad I did have a planned home birth, as I would have probably ended up giving birth in the car en route to the hospital.

I found the pushing stage quite overwhelming. I think I would have preferred to have used some gas and air at that point, but it all happened so quickly. I don't think either myself or the midwife were prepared for how fast he was going to arrive!

The stitching afterwards was quite painful, even more so than the labor. But once the local anaesthetic took effect and I'd sucked hard on the gas and air (which strangely tasted like amaretto), it was all floaty and fine.

What would you tell an expectant mother to better prepare her for childbirth?

Read up and look at the research and evidence, rather than just relying on online parenting forums. I researched VBACs and the associated risks in depth, and felt I was able to make a fully informed decision on my choice of care.

Trust your instincts. I felt that I would have a very quick labor, and so chose a planned home birth.

I used hypnobirthing and thoroughly recommend it! If you want to avoid using strong pain relief and all the associated risks, then this really enables you to let your mind relax and your body just get on with it. I feel it helped me have quick, easy labors.

I can only compare the active pushing stage to the vomiting reflex. Everyone is different, but I felt I had no control over my body at this stage. So the best thing to do is try and relax, instead of tensing up. When you get to this stage, it won't be long until you meet your baby!

So the best thing to do is try and relax, instead of tensing up. When you get to this stage, it won't be long until you meet your baby!

Kelly Price

Kelly shares with us the birth of her third child, which was her first birth at home. By birthing at home, Kelly had the most comfortable birth yet. She felt at ease and secure, but found some company and noise too intrusive. As relaxed as she may have been, she wishes her birth could have been even more peaceful. She reminds women to not fret if plans change, and encourages women to see childbirth as the beginning of new life.

The Birth of Jesse

*"It was the best experience of my life
and I wouldn't change it for the world."*

I gave birth to my third child and first boy at home, in the water, on April 30th, 2014. He was my first home birth and my first natural birth as well. I had my 40 week appointment with my midwife on my due date, and I was 4 cm and 75% effaced. I went home and was feeling a little crampy, but it was not consistent. Just before I went to bed at 11 pm, I texted my midwife to let her know.

That night, I was awoken at 3:30 am by a small contraction, which was followed by another. I realized that they were keeping me from sleeping, so I decided to get up and take a shower. Once in the washroom, I realized that I was bleeding, so I called my midwife. She told me to track my contractions for 30 minutes, and to let her know how far apart they were.

I jumped in the shower, but shortly after jumped out because I wanted to keep my hot water for the birthing pool. I told my husband that I was in labor, but insisted he continue sleeping, since it was his birthday.

I texted my midwife, Jessica, and told her my contractions were 10-12 minutes apart, lasting about 45 seconds. She had no plans that day and lived an hour away, so she decided to just come over. My close friend Brandi arrived after 4 am, followed by my midwife and her assistant. We talked, walked, and timed my contractions.

At 11 am, my contractions were 10 minutes apart. I was still at 4 cm, but now was 100% effaced. I took a cup of herbs to help make my contractions closer. We ordered pizza, laughed, and talked as the contractions got stronger and closer together.

To help move the baby down, and to assist in making my contractions more efficient, I squatted for every contraction. By about 2:30 pm, my contractions were between 5-8 minutes apart. They were much stronger, but I breathed through them all.

I was now at 7 cm, so we decided to get the pool ready. I bounced around on my birthing ball, and had nice conversations with everyone. While waiting for the pool to get ready, I laid on the bed, and had a few hard and long contractions. Around 3 pm, I went into transition, just as I was about to get into the pool. I got very emotional and started feeling a little lost. I started crying, but took a few deep breaths, and pulled myself together.

Once in the pool, I felt relieved that I was soon going to meet my son. The pool felt great and my contractions went back to being about 9-12 minutes apart.

Once in the pool, I felt relieved that I was soon going to meet my son.

I was still progressing great, and I was very relaxed. Around 3:45 pm, I started pushing, and at 4:08 pm, my beautiful son was born in the water. He was caught by his daddy, and put into the arms of his mommy. My daughters were riding their bikes outside with their grandmother, but came right in to meet their new baby brother. I was so relieved that it was over and that I was finally meeting my son for the first time.

My husband got out of the pool as I delivered the placenta. I had a bit of blurry vision due to pushing so hard, but I had no tears. I nursed about 30 minutes after he was born, and he latched right on like a pro.

Baby Jesse was a healthy and happy little man, weighing 8lbs 1oz, and was 20.5 inches long. He was born on his daddy's birthday, and shared his name.

Our family was there for about 2 hours after delivery. After they left, we were a family of five in the comfort of our own home. There is nothing like sleeping in your own bed only hours after giving birth. It was the best experience of my life and I wouldn't change it for the world.

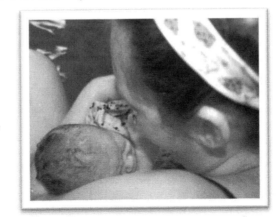

What did you like most about your childbirth experience?

What I liked most about my childbirth experience is the fact that I decided to give birth at home. I felt so comfortable being in my own space with all my own stuff. I wasn't getting poked and prodded the whole time, and I could eat whatever I wanted. My midwife was amazing and my birth team was great and extremely supportive. If I could go back, I would have birthed all my children at home.

What did you like least about your childbirth experience?

The thing I liked least about my childbirth experience was how noisy everyone was. If I could go back, I would have definitely asked everyone to be quieter. It was too loud when I was having contractions and right after he was born, there were so many conversations. My husband called the whole family and there were at least 20 people in my house minutes after our son was born. I felt a bit uncomfortable especially since I was having issues with my vision. I wish there would have been less people for my husband to have to occupy. I would have just wanted him by my side until everything was said and done, and I was dressed and ready to have people over.

What would you tell an expectant mother to better prepare her for childbirth?

Along with your birth plan, make sure you also state exactly how you want everything to go after the birth. For example, how and when to allow guests in, when you want to breastfeed, etc. When things don't go as planned, don't kick yourself, because this is labor. Things happen, and plans change. If plans fall through, that is OK. Childbirth is the first day of the rest of your life.

If plans fall through, that is OK. Childbirth is the first day of the rest of your life.

Kirrilee Heartman

Whether you are having your first child, or your fifth, Kirrilee's story shows you that each birth may be different. Your past experiences will affect the way you approach and think of childbirth. Despite negative memories, Kirrilee was able to allow her body to do what it does perfectly well on its own. She understood the important physiological parts of childbirth, and respected nature's gift. Her story teaches us that even though unexpected events may occur, you can remain calm and focused. Kirrilee encourages all women to embrace childbirth, and to prepare as best as they can for this incredible journey.

The Story of Robin's Birth

"All birthing women need to surrender themselves to the force of birth, for it to unfold smoothly."

Robin was my fifth baby, and my third home birth. As birthing time grew near, I felt myself slipping into a lovely connection with my family and with my midwife, as we had already been through two very different births together. As I went past 40 weeks, I was in no real hurry for the baby to come. I had lots of pre-labor sensations, but I knew it was just my body warming up. On the Sunday evening a week past the due date, I rang the midwife before bed, somehow feeling it was going to happen. In hindsight, I think I was already in the dreamy, detached, inward headspace of labor.

At 1:00 am, I woke with a strong contraction, and my waters had broken a little. I went to the loo only to realize that my perineum was completely swollen, and I felt that the baby had dropped down a lot. I didn't have very strong or regular contractions, but I woke Sol and told him to get the pool filled.

At 3:00 am, Sol told me to ring the midwife. I was reluctant as it was the middle of the night, but a suddenly stronger contraction gave me the sign I needed. She said she would just 'pop' over to have a look.

She arrived at 4:00 am, and after listening to the baby and sitting with me for a while, told me it was probably still early in the labor. However, the intensity picked up immediately after this, and I began having overwhelming contractions, for which I had to go deeply inward to focus through.

At 5:00 am, the midwife suggested I get into the pool after hearing me start to push. I said that I did not want to. In the last birth, I had felt a strong pain in my pelvis when the baby came through, and the memory of that difficult pain formed into a huge resistance now. I went to lie down, and all of a sudden she was there, rubbing my back and telling me it was all right. I said I was fed up with the contractions, and that I was scared of the pain. She said the baby would come anyway. Those few moments of tender words between just the two of us helped my resistance melt away.

I went to lie down, and all of a sudden she was there, rubbing my back and telling me it was all right.

I entered the pool. A couple of minutes in the water was enough to rejuvenate my spirits and to help me focus, ready for the second stage. After the second pushy contraction, there was a sudden popping sound. The outside of the pool had split down a seam! I sat up, the midwife swore, and Sol looked panicked. Time paused as we all looked at each other. Sol got a patch for the pool but when I leaned on it for the next contraction, it split again. The split was large enough to mean that we would have to abandon the water birth. Sol held the pool together while the midwife held my hand for another contraction, which didn't arrive. The labor had suddenly stalled. She and Sol began emptying the pool, but their nervous activity was beginning to affect me. I told them that they were freaking me out and took myself off to the loo for a while.

When I got back, the midwife had placed a towel over the lounge and on to the floor, so I went and knelt there. As soon as I did, the contractions started up again, and I felt the baby begin to move down. But no one was around – they were now madly bailing out the pool. The midwife, after hurriedly assuring me that she was still there for me, said we should wake up my mum and kids to help empty the pool.

Within a few minutes, I could feel the baby crowning. As that overwhelming urge to push came over me, I called for the midwife. As the baby's head emerged, I realized I didn't have that pelvic pain that I had experienced before, and that not being in the pool meant I could get in a better and more comfortable position for my body. I'd given one loud push, and then the midwife said to just breathe the baby out. I let go of the effort I was putting into pushing, and was amazed to feel his head just coming down on its own.

I knew that I didn't want to pause between head and body emerging. I gave myself permission to just keep nudging him out without stopping at all, and it felt like he slid out very easily and quickly. I think I went into a bit of shock, began crying and shaking, but also worrying that it had been too fast for me. As I turned around, I heard Sol exclaim 'Oh it's a boy!'

I was helped up to lay on the lounge - my mother and son were still bailing out the pool. My 12 year old son had been sitting two feet away from me as I gave birth, and my mum hadn't even realized the baby had come until I called her over to see him. He was born at 5:50 am and the placenta came quickly at 6 am. I ate a small piece raw – something I have done with every birth except one, as a symbolic act of giving back to my body, and as a measure to avoid excessive blood loss.

There were some magical moments when, at 7:00 am, the other kids all drifted out, sleepy-eyed, to find that the baby was finally here. Sol began preparing breakfast and the day began as usual. Despite the unexpected

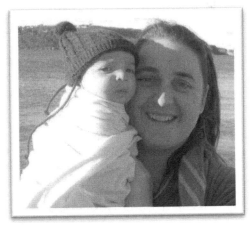

elements, it was a fantastic birth, easy on my body, and full of lightheartedness.

What did you like most about your childbirth experience?

What I liked the most about my childbirth experience was the ease I experienced, both physically when the baby was emerging, and emotionally. It was the easiest birth of all five. Home birth is very special in that birthing at home is seen as not special – it is an everyday occurrence and is left to unfold naturally at home.

> *Home birth is very special in that birthing at home is seen as not special – it is an everyday occurrence and is left to unfold naturally at home*

What did you like least about your childbirth experience?

What I liked least about my childbirth experience was the process of surrender. Having birthed many times, I know in detail what is going to happen and what it will feel like. In those final moments of birthing, I am present with the sensations, and am able to surrender to them and just flow. However, while in labor, especially with this fifth birth, I had a lot of resistance to the second stage. It was almost like I had to decide to do it, but the process took a while.

What would you tell an expectant mother to better prepare her for childbirth?

To prepare for childbirth, I recommend a few things. Firstly, know physically and physiologically what is going to happen, how the hormones act, and the different stages of childbirth.

Secondly, I think childbirth classes (not run by a hospital) are great. Classes that are aimed at supporting natural, active birth. I think it is important to acknowledge one's fears about birth while pregnant. I find a lot of journaling and meditation helpful here. Every night before sleeping, I also visualized, in detail, the birth I wished to experience. I really believe in the power of visualization, and have experienced five drug-free, completely unassisted, births.

For the actual birth, creating a safe space for the birthing mother is essential. It doesn't matter if it is at home or in a hospital. The environment can be made one's own. If the birthing mother does not feel safe, then how can her baby remain relaxed throughout the process? How can her body remain relaxed and let the baby out smoothly? The sense of safety applies to the immediate environment, lighting, people present and caregivers (this last point needs to be sorted out in pregnancy).

For the actual birth, creating a safe space for the birthing mother is essential.

Finally – the process I mentioned before: surrender. I think all birthing women need to surrender themselves to the force of birth, for it to unfold smoothly. Pain coping techniques help, and so does coming to a place of willingness to meet the baby. Do what needs to be done to get there!

Placenta Encapsulation: Mother Nature's Gift for Postpartum Wellness

Carmen Calvo

Having a baby can be a joyous occasion, but for some it can also be the cause of hormonal imbalances, which can result in a mother feeling emotions ranging from "the baby blues" to more serious forms of clinical depression. Mood imbalances are not uncommon among new mothers. In fact, 80% of new moms experience "the baby blues" and up to 20% suffer from postpartum depression.

In a study by The National Institute of Health, it was determined that the mid-pregnancy levels of Corticotropin-Releasing Hormone (CRH), a stress relieving hormone, may be an indicator of postpartum depression. CRH is typically produced by a part of the brain called the hypothalamus. However, during the 3rd trimester, the placenta produces so much CRH that the mother's levels increase threefold. This increase is thought to get her through the stress of labor and delivery. One result of the placenta secreting so much of this hormone is that the hypothalamus discontinues production of CRH completely.

Once the mother delivers the placenta, her hormone levels can go back to baseline within 5 days, resulting in a huge hormonal shift. It may take a few weeks after delivery for the hypothalamus to get the message that the baby has been born and mom is in need of CRH. It is during this gap between birth and when the body regulates itself that women typically experience the onset of postpartum mood disorders (PPMD).

Many antidepressants are a contraindication with breastfeeding, leaving some moms with the painful task of choosing between their own mental health and giving their baby the best start by breastfeeding.

Fortunately, there may be a holistic, more natural way to lessen a mother's risk factors for PPMD. Placenta, used for centuries in Traditional Chinese Medicine, may benefit a new mother's postpartum recovery. After delivery, the placenta retains many of the hormones that postpartum women are lacking. It is thought that by ingesting the placenta, also known as placentophagy, a mother can return to homeostasis more quickly. Typically considered medical waste in Western culture, the placenta can be used medicinally and has been reported to have a variety of benefits, including reducing one's risk for postpartum depression.

Placenta consumption may be unappetizing for some, but the process of placenta encapsulation can take the "ick" factor out of placentophagy. Placenta encapsulation, the process of turning your baby's placenta into capsules, can be consumed like any other supplement or vitamin. The process, performed by a trained professional, takes about 2 days and consists of cleaning the placenta, gently steaming it using Traditional Chinese methods, and preparing it for dehydration. Once the placenta is dried, it can be pulverized and made into capsules.

By ingesting the placenta and her own hormones, a postpartum mom may be able to experience the following:

ENHANCED LACTATION:

Prolactin, a hormone contained in the placenta, is necessary for milk production. In one study of 210 women, 86% had an increase in milk production when given dried placenta vs. a dried beef alternative.

INCREASED ENERGY AND LESS FATIGUE:

It's no surprise new mothers are tired. Their sleep schedules are often interrupted, they are nursing their new baby around the clock, and they are adjusting to their new role as a mother. However, fatigue may also be due to iron deficiency in postpartum mothers. It has been identified that iron deficiency can play a role in the onset of PPD. The placenta is loaded with natural iron and can be very beneficial to postpartum moms. Since the iron contained in the placenta is in its natural state, it is more easily absorbed by the mother.

A BALANCED MOOD, DECREASED RISK OF PPMD:

By reintroducing mom's hormones, she is more likely to avoid the severe hormonal fluctuations many postpartum women face. The placenta is full of hormones, minerals, and vitamins; even after parturition. Prolactin, oxytocin, estrogen, estriol, CRH, and thyroid-releasing hormone are only a few of the beneficial hormones a mother can consume when ingesting her placenta.

DECREASED POSTNATAL BLEEDING:
Placenta encapsulation may help a mother's uterus contract back to normal size more quickly, which can hasten postpartum bleeding. Placing a piece of raw placenta between a hemorrhaging mother's gum and cheek can be a very helpful tool for controlling excessive bleeding after birth.

While the anecdotal evidence of the benefits of placenta encapsulation is overwhelming, research on placentophagy is still very much in its infancy. It is, however, encouraging that interest in the topic is growing. Last year, University of Nevada, Las Vegas released a scholarly report on placenta consumption in postpartum mothers.

The findings were that 96% had a positive experience consuming their placenta and 98% would do it again if they had another baby. A peer reviewed placebo vs. placenta study is currently taking place at UNLV and the results should be reported in the next 2 years.

Hopefully, when the study is published, we will be able to gain a deeper understanding of how placenta encapsulation benefits a postpartum mother.

To learn more about placenta encapsulation or to find a specialist in your area, visit placentabenefits.info.

Carmen Calvo is a Certified Placenta Encapsulation Specialist and Birth Boot Camp Instructor in Baltimore, MD. Shortly after the birth of her second child in 2011, Carmen started The Nurturing Root and began offering placenta encapsulation services. After achieving a balanced and good postpartum experience through placenta encapsulation, Carmen felt inspired to help other women in her community achieve the same. You can email her at carmen@thenurturingroot.com or visit her website at www.thenurturingroot.com.

Kayla Suderman

Kayla's birth story shows us that labor is not a stagnant point in time. Labor can change and shift direction. The course of labor is influenced by the expectant mother, and by her environment. Knowing this, expectant moms can better understand their role in childbirth. It is not simply something that 'happens to them.' Childbirth is influenced by many factors, and at the same time it also influences a variety of other elements. From Kayla's story, we learn that as technologically advanced as we may be, life will never cease to amaze us. Or surprise us.

The Birth of Bree

"It was a startling, yet amazing, feeling."

Wednesday around 9 pm, I started having contractions that seemed like "this was it." For several weeks, I'd experienced prodromal labor and was emotionally exhausted from all the false starts. I was apprehensive to admit this was actual labor. Hubby, however, noticed a change in my behavior and called our midwife around 10:30 pm to let her know things had begun.

Around midnight, our midwife arrived. Her assistant followed 10 minutes later. My good friend Casey had already arrived as our doula and photographer, and was sitting and chatting with us. I spent the whole evening pacing the floors and walking the stairs through contractions. My contractions were 3 minutes apart and 1 minute long, though still tolerable. Around 1 am, I was 6-7 cm dilated. This made me hopeful that labor would be short, as transition was just around the corner, and active labor had been almost "too easy" up to that point. I was able to still walk through contractions, though talking was becoming less easy. I was enjoying the company of my labor support team, something I was unable to do with my first birth due to extremely intense back labor.

Unfortunately, I started questioning whether this was going anywhere because it was much easier than my first birth. I worried this was the worst prodromal labor yet, and allowed myself to panic. Though my contractions remained 3 minutes apart and 1 minute long, they stopped growing in intensity. By 3 am Thursday, it was obvious things had stalled. At 6 am, my midwife asked if I was OK with them going to grab something for breakfast. Hubby and I took the opportunity to sleep, in hopes that rest would allow my body to resume what it was trying to do.

At 8 am, I shot awake. I had several contractions in a row that were too intense for me to relax. I felt nauseous. I called hubby into the living room, and right as he came in, I threw up into a bowl that was on the coffee table. I did a lousy job of keeping myself calm. I kept asking for my midwife. Then I started crying and said I was scared. Hubby reminded me this was a sign of the end and that he was proud of me. His encouragement was enough to calm me until our birth team arrived.

His encouragement was enough to calm me until our birth team arrived.

Casey immediately started bath water for me, as I wanted a water birth. I paced the house between contractions and stopped to moan through them. I anxiously waited to jump into that hot water! Once my body hit the hot water, I felt the tension melt away. The next few contractions were decreased in intensity so much I smiled through them, munched on a peach fruit bar, and sipped water.

For the next 2 1/2 hours, I labored in the tub. I sat and rocked my hips, or leaned into a crouching position to rock my hips. Around 11 am, my midwife said to stand and to put a leg on the side of the tub for the next 5-6 contractions. The intensity of pain that the water had masked came back, and I recognized it as true transition. My midwife clutched my head to her chest during contractions and breathed along with me to keep me calm. She then had me face her directly and hang on her shoulders during contractions. It was then I felt the urge to bear down. The contractions I felt this labor were entirely different than what I experienced the first time. These were low in my abdomen and focused right around the cervix. The force of the cramps made me very aware I was dilating, and the more I focused on dilating the more I started to feel the head move lower. It was a startling, yet amazing, feeling.

At 9 cm, we discovered the bag of water bulging in front of the head. Both my midwife and I tried pinching it to break it, but it was too strong. I switched positions instead to give the baby more room to move. Reclined against the tub, I was able to start pushing the head into the birth canal. Once I felt the head enter the birth canal, the bag of water popped. As I was delivering the head, I instinctively got onto my knees and after several big pushes, our baby slipped gracefully into the water.

At our ultrasound, we had been told we were having a boy and though we revealed the gender to everyone we decided to keep the name a secret until his birth. Immediately, our birth team asked what his name was. I blurted out, "Haddon!" It felt great to finally say his name to others! The next thing that escaped my lips was a huge gasp. I was staring not at a penis but a vagina! There was a moment of utter silence. Stunned, I reclined against the tub and vacantly stared into space for a few seconds. Hubby just laughed. We both were in disbelief.

Hubby just laughed. We both were in disbelief.

Almost 48 hours later, we settled on a name: Bree Gracelyn. She arrived at 40 weeks, 4 days at 8lbs 10 oz, and 21 inches long.

Unfortunately, I did have a postpartum hemorrhage. I had no tearing, swelling or bruising from delivery, so it was discouraging to deal with a hemorrhage since my labor and delivery otherwise had been wonderful. My midwife dealt with it quickly by giving me a shot of Pitocin and doing fundal massage. I'm so thankful for our home birth, and grateful for such skilled midwives who are calm in the face of complications, and supportive during one of the most important moments of our lives. And of course the arrival of our surprise daughter made it an even more unforgettable memory!

What did you like most about your childbirth experience?

I loved the quietness of a home birth. It was such a nice contrast to the busy hospital birth I had with our first child. I was never interrupted, prodded, forced to sign waivers during hard contractions, and I was free to eat, drink, and move about as I wanted. It felt so normal to just be home and give birth. Afterwards, both my husband and I felt relaxed and at peace, unlike our hospital birth where we both struggled with depression and stress for weeks following the birth.

I loved the quietness of a home birth. It was such a nice contrast to the busy hospital birth I had with our first child.

What did you like least about your childbirth experience?

There was nothing I disliked about my home birth experience!

What would you tell an expectant mother to better prepare her for childbirth?

Know what YOU want for your birth and how YOU want to experience it. Then, find a supportive care provider. Remember your care provider is HIRED by you, so if you're unimpressed with their service or attitude towards your wants, fire them and find someone else. Few people would allow a home remodeler to criticize their home and then remodel it how THEY wanted, while disrespecting your desires. If a house is worth standing up for, how much more important is your body?

Sally Lansdale

Sally's childbirth took place in the 1970s, but remains very relevant to today's birth culture. As you read it, you may realize that not much has changed over the past forty years. Many women continue to face various obstacles preventing them from having the childbirth that they would like. Even though she was a single mother, Sally had a support system that helped her feel secure and comfortable during this period. Sally understood that childbirth was a precious time, which should not be over-medicalized. She knew what she wanted, and did everything she could to make it as special as possible.

The Birth of Seth

"It was a joyful, happy day. I was in a safe and loving place."

My name is Sally Lansdale. It was December 1975, when it became clear I was pregnant. I was 23, and in a new relationship. I wasn't sure if the relationship was going anywhere, but when I told him I was pregnant, had I been completely objective at the time, it would have been clear that the relationship was going nowhere. He was not ready. He had plans. He was moving north to Monterey to attend Chiropractic College. He was going. He was gone. I only saw him a couple of times after that.

I went over all options in my head; adoption, abortion, motherhood. I went over all the things I had done versus all the things I hadn't done but wanted to. I decided I could live without ever jumping a freight train and opted for motherhood.

From the very beginning of this pregnancy, I was a single mother. But I wasn't on my own. I had a close circle of friends who were likeminded. I had a ton of support. My family was amazingly supportive.

My first prenatal visit was at UCLA, where a young resident examined me. It was obvious he was not familiar with what he was feeling. He called in his teacher. He gloved up, poked around and immediately said, "Wow! You have a HUGE pelvis!" I knew I would have no problems giving birth.

Many of my friends were young mothers. Most of them had given birth "naturally" using either the Lamaze or Bradley childbirth "methods," and some had given birth at home. After some research, I decided Dr. Bradley's method made more sense to me, and found a teacher and a coach. At my first class, the teacher talked about the importance of having an advocate in the hospital. She indicated that hospital workers will assume you want pain medication, and thus will continually offer it to you. She coached the husbands on how to be strong advocates for their wives while dealing with hospital staff.

I didn't have a husband. I had a good friend and coach, but I didn't have a husband to speak for me.

I was referred to Nial B. Ettinghausen, D.P.[9] He was licensed as a Drugless Practitioner (specializing in childbirth at home) in 1939, and as a Chiropractor in 1942. I read about childbirth in England where drugs were not part of the deal, where lying flat on your back in a brightly lit operating theater was not the norm. I was already alone as a single mother-to-be. I wanted to give birth where I felt safe, protected, and loved.

I wanted to give birth where I felt safe, protected, and loved.

I immediately trusted Dr. Ettinghausen, a gentle man, about the same age as my father. He confirmed that I seemed to have the right bone structure for an easy birth. I lived in Redondo Beach, a long drive from his office, but he had a group of nurse-midwives on his staff that worked in pre-arranged sectors of the Los Angeles area. One would be assigned to me and would stay with me from start to finish.

My child was due to be born the first part of July. At most of my visits, Dr. E. would listen for a second heartbeat while I held my breath. In June, he became concerned that we had miscalculated my due date. Did I remember my dates

---

[9] http://www.gentlebirth.org/format/ettinghausen.html

correctly? I did. In fact, I had become pregnant no earlier than October; I knew because it had been the first time with my young man. Nonetheless, Dr. E. wanted to be sure there weren't two fetuses in there, and recommended I have an X-Ray. Seriously? He assured me it would be safer to have one X-Ray than not to.

The X-Ray confirmed one beautiful child, facing the right direction, head perfectly positioned. One tiny little spine, nestled safely in the shelter of my larger one.

When calculating the due date using the date of the last period and counting back two weeks, my due date was July 8th. My mother said, "Add two weeks to whatever they tell you."

My roommate went out of town the weekend of July 17th. If I went into labor, I was to immediately call her boyfriend and he would come over. I woke up around 1 am on the 18th with a backache. It took me a while to figure it out. I called the boyfriend. He was probably terrified, but he came over and stayed there while I drifted in and out of sleep.

Sunday morning came and I called my friend Terri, who was my birth coach, and Dr. E's answering service. The nurse-midwife, a woman named Dorothy, whose last name I never recorded, came along with a young woman, Dr. Cheryl Harder, who was studying under Dr. E. for the summer. They set up shop with a table (Dr. E's knees could no longer handle bed births), a scale to weigh the baby, and what else, I couldn't tell you; I was busy. Dr. Harder made herbal tea. Dr. E popped in and out during the long day. At his last visit he was dressed in suit and tie, on his way to give a lecture on home birth. If I still hadn't had the baby when he came back, he would break my water to move things along.

My coach helped me to relax my toes, my fingers, and my eyebrows. She leaned on my back while I was on my knees, with my head on the sofa to relieve the back labor. She walked with me around my block all afternoon. She held my knees back while I pushed. After 45 minutes of pushing, with the last three

After 45 minutes of pushing, with the last three pushes to get his broad shoulders loose, he entered our world.

pushes to get his broad shoulders loose, he entered our world.

Seth was born at 7:47 pm, on July 18th, 1976 as the red rays of sunset shone in my window. He weighed 11lbs 2oz and was 22 inches long. When Dr. E. checked back around 10 pm, he turned on the light and the baby cried. He picked up the baby, stroked his head, and he quieted right down.

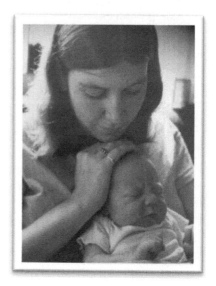

The next morning, my sister arrived, my roommate got back from her trip, and I had a nice breakfast of cantaloupe and strawberries while I nursed my big, happy, sweet, baby boy.

That boy is 6' 4" of manhood now, with five children of his own.

What did you like most about your childbirth experience?

It was a joyful, happy day. I was in a safe and loving place. I didn't have to get in a car and drive across town while in labor. I didn't have to deal with strangers, or have an advocate to insist I not be strapped down and given an epidural... or Valium.

My second child was 9lbs 10oz, and I was chatting with the midwives and my birth coach all the way up to the last push.

What did you like least about your childbirth experience?

The table, but I almost forgot that I was disappointed to have to use it. I didn't have any desire to go on my hands and knees. I had support behind my back, and someone held each leg by the knee, so I could give birth reclined rather than squatting.

What would you tell an expectant mother to better prepare her for childbirth?

Read Dr. Bradley's book. If you can find it, read Dr. Ettinghausen's book, "Skilled Childbirth At Home" (1975) in paperback by Dr. Nial Ettinghausen D.C., D.P., revised and re-published as "Childbirth at Its Best" (1980) in hardback.

After the birth of my second child, at home, my cervix started to close up before the placenta was born. The midwife gave me a shot of Pitocin. Giving birth to the placenta was harder than giving birth to the child.

Finally, if you must use a hospital, *switch doctors* if he/she informs you they are going to induce you if you go past your due date. It's a load of crap to make the doctor's life easier.

Switch doctors if he/she informs you they are going to induce you if you go past your due date. It's a load of crap to make the doctor's life easier.

The Over-Medicalization of Childbirth

Marika Jeziorek

>*"The interpretation and discourse of childbirth needs to be deconstructed, to reveal all of its flaws and misunderstandings, and built anew, as a completely natural phenomenon that women can undergo without (unnecessary) intervention or abuse." – Marika Jeziorek*

SAVING LIVES IN CHILDBIRTH

It remains a tragedy that hundreds of thousands of women and newborns around the world continue to die from pregnancy-related complications and unsanitary conditions. It is a global responsibility that we have ignored and prefer to continue ignoring. But even though it may be deadly at times, childbirth remains a normal biological phenomenon.

Medical advancement, such as obstetrics, has been tremendously helpful in saving lives. But as Johanson et al. explain, the decrease in maternal and newborn mortality must also be attributed to overall advances in developed countries, such as healthcare and disease control, higher standards of living, smaller family sizes, and improved diet. To understand the decrease in maternal and newborn mortality, one must consider all factors involved, including indirect causes and effects.

Even though these lower mortality rates are a result of a combination of variables, we have carefully selected medical advancement as the leading source of better maternal care and fewer lost lives. As a result, medical intervention has become routine, without evidence of effectiveness (Johanson et al.). In many cases, medical assistance and medical practice has become the most valued component in labor and delivery.

In her article "Why is Childbirth a Medical Procedure?," Dr. Earle explains that the majority of women in the UK are subjected to a magnitude of medical and technological interventions throughout their pregnancy and birth. During labor, women with straightforward pregnancies are subjected to routine infusions and oxytocin, are regularly given epidurals, are systematically under electronic fetal monitoring, and are encouraged to labor and deliver in the lying down position (Johanson et al.). Because of these preferred practices, labor intervention, assisted delivery (i.e. forceps, vacuums), and major surgery (C-sections) have become widespread. These interventions have led to even more repercussions, including painful intercourse and urinary and anal incontinence (Johanson et al.). Dr. Earle argues that "the routine medicalization of childbirth robs women, midwives, and society, of the knowledge and experience of what it is to have a normal birth."

> *We have succumbed to whatever the medical establishment prefers and advocates, in the belief that it will continue to save and help the lives that it does, regardless of any possible side-effects.*

Despite medical intervention and the medical environment not being the sole determinants in maternal and newborn health, we have succumbed to whatever the medical establishment prefers and advocates, in the belief that it will continue to save and help the lives that it does, regardless of any possible side-effects.

STEP 1: ADMIT THERE IS A PROBLEM

But we know there is a problem. A very big problem. When surveyed, 51% of obstetricians in England, Wales, and Northern Ireland expressed concern that their C-section rates were too high (Paranjothy). Johanson et al. explain that pregnant women continue to be silenced and considered irrelevant in decision making. This abuse and disrespect continues around the world.

Since it has been established that we are in fact, over-medicalizing childbirth in countries that are privileged enough to call themselves 'developed', it is time to question why we are experiencing this need to control and create technologically-dependent solutions to problems that may not even exist. Why are we so dependent on (unnecessary) medical intervention, especially during such a natural event like childbirth?

STEP 2: DO SOMETHING ABOUT IT

Top-Down Approach

So what can be done to bring back childbirth to its original understanding, as a normal part of life, where women are not subjected to the calculated treatment that is preferred by medical professionals?[10] Where they believe in their own ability to birth, without intervention or special equipment? Let us first look at the top-down, from the higher-ups, approach to rethinking childbirth.

Countries that pride themselves over low intervention rates (i.e. the Scandinavian countries and the Netherlands), and those that have not been eager to implement birth interventions, define childbirth as a normal physiological process (Paranjothy). Beginning in the early 20th century, the low maternal mortality present in the Netherlands, Norway, and Sweden was attributed to a close collaboration between obstetricians and highly competent midwives (De Brouwere et al.). This comprehensive understanding of childbirth, as requiring not only medical assistance if needed, but also one-on-one emotional and physical support, has been shown to achieve exceptional results.

To help de-medicalize childbirth, the Ontario Women's Health Council has previously suggested the following items: to foster an understanding of childbirth as a normal physiological process, to encourage a sense of pride when hospitals have low C-section rates, and to provide one-on-one support to women in labor. Similarly, the Expert Advisory Group on Caesarean Section in Scotland has encouraged a systematic review of C-section rates, one-on-one midwifery support for every woman in

---

[10] The preferred medical practice and procedures that may result of convenience, understanding, or fear of blame.

labor, as well as other evidence-based recommendations. Change is happening.

It is time to reconsider the role of intervention and standard routine practices that have led to serious ramifications for mothers and their babies. Women need to be respected and supported to labor and deliver in a dignified and gentle way. But a refined collaboration between obstetricians and midwives, and a new understanding by medical professionals, is not enough. We also need to help guide a more positive cultural understanding and perception of childbirth.

Bottom-Up Approach

Re-organizing the birthing unit and the mentality of healthcare providers, to present childbirth in a more positive light, combined with a cultural-based approach, can do wonders. Let us now look at the bottom-up (grassroots) approach to creating a positive and gentle understanding of childbirth.

Books, movies, blogs, documentaries, etc. are being produced and shared far and wide, through neighbors, friends, and social media profiles. Gratitude needs to be expressed to Ina May Gaskin, Pam England, Ricki Lake, and other big and small personalities for their contribution to helping shape the perception of childbirth into a more peaceful and joyful one.

Social advocates of peaceful and empowered childbirth are stripping away the layers of false accusations and stereotypes, and bringing to light the reality that (most) women are strong and absolutely capable of giving birth without intervention. These advocates understand the repercussions of portraying women as helpless beings who are only capable of lying on a bed with lights up their vagina. These advocates are reminding women that this

> *These advocates understand the repercussions of portraying women as helpless beings who are only capable of lying on a bed with lights up their vagina.*

can be done. They can have a voice in deciding how they give birth, where they give birth, and with whom they give birth. Decision-making is attainable for women. Advocates are fighting for the right of women to influence their childbirth. To be important actors during this transition into motherhood.

Perhaps most importantly, there is a growing number of expectant moms grasping the resources they need to achieve the childbirth that they want. They are learning the various techniques, methods, and tools that they can use to achieve a peaceful home, hospital, or birthing center birth. They are demanding midwifery care when there is none. They are lobbying and standing up against violence in obstetrics and childbirth. They are sharing stories and providing wisdom to others, with the hope of alleviating fear and encouraging strength. Women are empowering themselves, and fighting for their rights in childbirth.

A DUAL APPROACH TO REINVENTING CHILDBIRTH

Combining a top-down and bottom-up approach to reinventing childbirth can provide the most amount of success. When the medical establishment understands the need to respect women in childbirth, and to not push for unnecessary interventions, we are developing a dignified and safe birthing environment for women. When the healthcare system understands the vital role of midwives in childbirth, then we are providing a nurturing and supportive environment for women where they see themselves as important decision makers influencing their birth. When our culture begins to understand childbirth as a natural and joyful event that can absolutely be empowering and incredible, we are alleviating common fear, anxiety, and doubt. When mothers educate themselves on the best techniques and methods, and when they demand the care that they want, we are developing a new generation of women and mothers who value their worth and who want to take control of their birth. When we combine all of these factors, we are reinventing childbirth into something special. Something that is understood in a positive light, where women can experience great joy, power, and strength.

Though she has produced an extensive array of articles during her undergraduate and graduate studies, "True Birth" is Marika's first book. She is a strong advocate of gentle parenting practices, women's and children's rights, and overall international development. You can see more of her work at www.FeelGoodGivingBirth.com, www.JCGrowth.com, and www.MomsTwoHourWorkDay.com.

Sources

De Brouwere V, Tonglet R, Van Lerberghe W. "Strategies for reducing maternal mortality in developing countries: what can we learn from the history of the industrialized West?" *Trop Med Int Health.* 1998 Oct; 3(10):771-82.

Earle, Sarah. "Why is Childbirth a Medical Procedure?" *The Open University.* 19 May 2005.

Expert Advisory Group on Caesarean Section in Scotland. Scottish programme for clinical effectiveness in reproductive health. Edinburgh: Clinical Resorce and Audit Group, Scottish Executive Health Department; 2001.

Johanson, Richard, Mary Newborn, and Alison Macfarlane. "Has the medicalization of childbirth gone too far?" *British Medical Journal* 324. 13 April 2002.

Ontario Women's Health Council. "Attaining and maintaining best practices in the use of caesarean sections." Toronto, Ontario: Ontario Women's Health Council; 2000.

Paranjothy S, Thomas J. Royal College of Obstetricians and Gynaecologists Clinical Effectiveness Support Unit. National sentinel caesarean section audit report. London: RCOG Press; 2001.

Avanya

Remember to expect the unexpected. Despite being past her EDD, Avanya did not worry. Her story depicts the raw power that shines when a woman is giving birth naturally. 'Labor land' as some would call it. Instead of fearing it, and sheepishly giving up, she embraced what was happening, and held her own. Even though the unexpected happened, Avanya is proud to have given birth, and encourages all women to realize just how strong they really are.

The Birth of Andy

"The beauty and the victory in reaching that mountaintop is as fresh to me today as it was that night."

I'd never gone more than two days past my due date. By the time I was a week past my due date with Andy, I was near hysterics. I'd woken up several nights with strong contractions, and paced the downstairs rooms in a slow rhythm, swaying my hips. There were contraction timers and watchful eyes, waiting for more. Then, the contractions would fade with the night, I'd return to bed, and my labor would sleep with me. For three nights the same thing, and still nothing.

Finally, I woke up with noticeable tightening. It was a holiday and my husband stayed home from work. He drove me to the chiropractor, then I insisted on buying new soap to use for my shower after the birth. I always love that shower after the ordeal of labor. He raised his eyebrows a bit and we bought soap. Coming home, I folded laundry, stopping at contractions, and then continuing on with my work. Soon, I could no longer walk through each wave, and acquiesced to calling my midwife. I remember clearly explaining "the shape of my hill is changing. I'm climbing mountains now." I think it was after that phrase that she came over, although I never asked.

I didn't want to seem over eager and was so concerned that I was imagining things. It was such an odd feeling to have my midwives arrive and still be unsure if it was really labor? Smiling and calm, they set up their supplies.

It went on for hours. In the bathtub, the moaning, the waiting, and the knowing that another one was coming. Hoping someone will crack a joke to distract you, and the pain when they do, and you laugh.

Then my children had their pajamas on, and darkness fell. Wasn't it just morning? Where was the baby? I really didn't think I was imagining that I was in labor, but what if? Someone, talk to me, distract me. No, leave me be. Wondering with each wave, is this the one? Do I need to push? Finally, I looked in my midwife's eyes, and said yes, at the tail end, yes. A hint that it would come, not the real feeling of a push. She nods, knowing. I realize how loud I am. I'm roaring. Holding my hand isn't helping at all, but please, don't let go. I don't even know whose hand it is, just please, don't let go.

> *Finally, I looked in my midwife's eyes, and said yes, at the tail end, yes.*

Suddenly, I hear POP! Who heard that? I see my husband getting nervous, like I've really lost my mind now. My mentors know. It's OK, we didn't hear it. It must be your water releasing! So close now. I can't catch my breath as the waves overtake me. I am helpless, at their mercy, spaghetti with the power of the universe behind me. I feel my legs cramping from holding my muscles so taut but I can't bear to move. Then it won't stop...I roar as before but the train pushes forward and there's no stopping. I cannot breathe and must GET THIS OUT OF ME, but it's impossible. I cannot do it and someone must help me! Somehow, this tiny, leftover fiber of strength rises up. I lean back on my husband's legs. The head must be out. I cannot do more. Someone says, "The head is almost out!" and I think ALMOST? Then, the calm words with eye contact and firm voice, the instructions. I have nothing left, they are saying "push, it is right here." I don't look away, but suddenly everything is fast. I know something is not right and someone else is guiding. I am grateful and I'm moving? How? Who stood me up? Is there not a head between my legs? Holding my hand, eye contact, calm words, firm voice. They can handle this, that's all I can understand. My leg is up. Who is holding my leg? Then GUSH and WHOOSH and I **GRAB** and my baby is in my arms! How? How? He's here! Don't let me go I don't want to fall! He is here. Perfect. He looks at my husband over my shoulder, eyes wide. He's here.

Later, I learn that his head was sideways. He was OK, but that was hard. He came out staring straight to my left, making mama work for every inch. My midwives, always with me, telling me yes, all was well, but you had spent all you had. You needed to stand so he could slide out and you couldn't, so we did it for you. I did realize that, but I was so foggy. For you it was, they say, but we are always there, always watching, always with you. You just needed to let gravity work. My indebtedness knows no bounds.

I lay on my bed and hold my baby. My husband holds me. My mother watches on. I'm told my children are well. One asleep, too young to hang on to the late night. My daughter, always by me, waiting right outside, happy to see me smile. And at last I shower, alone again.

Birthing Andy was like climbing a mountain, using every ounce of strength and then a bit more. The beauty and the victory in reaching that mountaintop is as fresh to me today as it was that night.

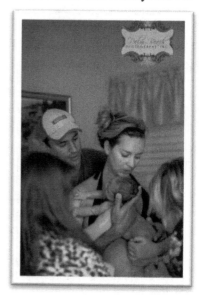

There's a spot of blood still on the door of my bathroom. I couldn't wash it. That smudge was full of so much strength. I showed my sister once, and explained. She nodded, knowing. That blood is precious, it birthed your son. Today, watching him play with his brother and sister while I cleaned up, scrubbing the dirt of yesterday to make room for the dirt of today, I saw that smudge. In an instant I washed it away. It's in my heart now. I fought for you, my son. I bled for you. I birthed you with great pain, and it is healed with the sight of your smile.

What did you like most about your childbirth experience?

There are many things that I liked about my birth, but I think what made the biggest impact on me was the atmosphere of strength. Normally I prefer to be alone, and have often said that if I could, I would birth alone in a closet and just let my husband know when I was done. For various reasons, there were quite a few people present for this birth, and while that was my choice, I expected to be a little uncomfortable with that aspect. Instead, I fed off their strength. The attentiveness of the midwives to my health, mental state, physical needs, and the anticipation of what was next was incomparable. They were calm but confident in my abilities. Every time I got to a point of doubt, there was a woman there with a hand or word to push me on.

Every time I got to a point of doubt, there was a woman there with a hand or word to push me on.

What did you like least about your childbirth experience?

It's difficult to say that something was disliked. Everything that happened that I could control, I did. The only time anyone else made a suggestion, or guided the process was when I had no strength left, and I was so thankful for it! Of course the length of labor, twelve hours, was frustrating, especially being much longer than my most recent labor. But I can't dislike that, it's just "an is," as my midwife says.

What would you tell an expectant mother to better prepare her for childbirth?

If I were telling an expectant mother something important, it would be that you will be OK. You will live. You will birth this baby, and you will feel proud of yourself for that. Somehow, I think that fundamental knowledge makes all the difference. Also, to look forward to what birth will do to you as a person. It will fundamentally change how you see yourself, and you should take great pride in knowing you birthed a child, no matter how hard or easy you perceive it to have been, or what the circumstances surrounding the details are. The idea of this seems impossible ahead of time, and then shortly after, seems to fade a bit. I wish that weren't the case. Think about and live in that proud, conquering mentality, and try to apply it to the other aspects of your life. I often repeat to myself "I birthed a baby in a bathtub, I can do this too." I think approaching labor as a challenging but rewarding personal experience, with a definite ending, has helped me immensely during the labor process!

> *You should take great pride in knowing you birthed a child, no matter how hard or easy you perceive it to have been, or what the circumstances surrounding the details are.*

Amaris Jitaru

Our last story is absolutely incredible. The author shows women that birth can be beautiful. It can be peaceful. Even joyful. Amaris believes that the location and the environment of the birth will influence how you experience this milestone. Having birthed in a hospital twice before, Amaris realized she was missing an important component: intimacy. Despite being a medical professional, she decided to birth at home for her youngest daughter. This is her story.

Serafina's Birth Story

"Do not be afraid of it, embrace each contraction
as life-giving force with which to birth your child."

When I was twenty-six, I met my true love. Within two weeks of our marriage we were expecting identical twin boys. An international move, precarious finances, mingled with the fear instilled in us at every medical appointment, made it that my first birth was a Caesarean Section. The sweet bitterness was made more tolerable by an act of fate or God's mercy- I went into labor the night of my scheduled C-section. Maybe it was out of dread.

Two years later, now well into my medical residency, I had a triumphant but painful VBAC in the hospital where I worked. After successfully laboring at home with my doula for many hours, my labor immediately stalled in the hospital for over ten hours. Had I been less informed, I would have been another surgical victim of Freidman's Curve.

Although my VBAC was empowering and healing, I found both of my hospital births were lacking something. The fundamental element missing was intimacy. With my third pregnancy, I plotted, and schemed, and read extensively.

It was a Tuesday afternoon and I had come home just that morning from a 24-hour hospital call. Around 3 **pm**, I mentioned to my husband that I was having some rather persistent contractions. Around 7 pm, I called my doula and midwife so they would rest. By 9 pm, I had showered and cuddled in bed next to my husband and the kids. I was having to concentrate more and more on my breathing and found it quite uncomfortable to sit still in bed.

I took my husband to our spare bedroom to begin the work of more intense labor together, in a room full of roses and candles. We drank sweetened lavender tea and swayed together in the harmonious rhythm of this natural birth, this celebration, this feast of life. Looking into each other's eyes, we exchanged joy and sentiments of profundity and intimacy that only we would know – we, who had participated in the creation of the soul about to be born.

We drank sweetened lavender tea and swayed together in the harmonious rhythm of this natural birth, this celebration, this feast of life.

I had explored my fears and misgivings throughout 9 months, so that the night of Serafina's birth, I felt only tremendous strength and readiness. I knew I was safe because I was where I felt the safest and was surrounded by love. I recall my youngest boy waking up around 1 am, shortly after my doula had arrived, and me nursing him back to sleep as I labored to bring his new sister into the world. We spoke together about how the baby was preparing to come.

I began to feel the need to go deep within myself. Because I started the labor on my own, with my husband, I did not feel the need to involve my doula physically as I had done with my previous birth. As the pain of the contractions increased slowly and naturally, I learned to receive it and work with it to birth my baby. Most of my intense labor was from 2 am onwards, and I spent my time standing and rocking, crouching and groaning, grabbing arms and pushing into my husband. My midwife and her assistant arrived about 2:30 am, and in the calmest, most natural way made themselves comfortable in our tiny room, dozing off to the primeval music of my labored groans.

If I had advice about how to deal with this pain naturally, I would say - do not be afraid of it, embrace each contraction as life-giving force with which to birth your child. I envisioned myself opening during these surges, and instead of retreating and contracting, I relaxed and allowed nature to do its millenary work.

At some point, there came a time when I knew I was almost ready for the baby to come, as the pain had reached a very intense level, and contractions were long and deep. My midwife and I agreed to break the sac of waters, as we both knew at almost full dilation, it was the only thing keeping me from pushing the baby. I braced myself for that indescribable urge that is so much beyond words. A minute or two must have passed after the water broke, and then it came: immense, ravishing, like an ocean of heavy water rising in its entirety to the heavens and crashing back down into its cove. I heaved and pushed, half rising from my birth stool with such a loud scream that I could have shook the walls of Jericho and I did not stop until I held Serafina in my arms. I remember vague voices pleading me to stop but I also remember that I simply could not. I thought during those moments, if you can call it thinking, that even if my body was torn in half and I was left tattered in shreds, I could not stop.

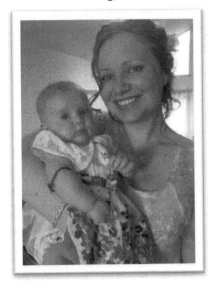

At 4:55 in the morning, an hour from the dawn of day, our little girl was born, small and slippery, perfectly shaped and wondrously made. She was welcomed into the world by her mother's warm, trembling arms, her father's tearful, starlit eyes and the midwife's glorious exclamation "Praised be the Lord!" The rest

occurred as would in a home birth, with patience, and skill, and love. Serafina nursed immediately. The afterbirth was allowed to come naturally; I cut her cord about an hour after our birth. I was laid as a queen on my bed and my three boys, now awake and alight with curiosity and excitement, inspected every aspect of the afterbirth. We entered our herbal bath together, mother and baby and babies. And, after we had bathed, we cuddled and talked, and ate a homestead breakfast. We fell soundly asleep; a family of five now made into six, with Serafina taking her place so naturally in bed among the boys.

What did you like most about your childbirth experience?

The familiarity and comfort of home where I was surrounded in a natural way by my husband and children. I didn't have to worry about touching the sterile field by mistake. I loved the dim lighting. I loved that I was left to labor however I wanted with no restrictions. There were no threats and there was no pressure to perform. This, and the safety I felt, led to relaxation, and that in turn helped the birth process enormously. The stress and anxiety of the unfamiliar place, people, and procedures of the hospital are some of the most detrimental things in hospital births.

This, and the safety I felt, led to relaxation, and that in turn helped the birth process enormously.

What did you like least about your childbirth experience?

There was nothing I did not like. I liked my bathroom, my shower, my mug of water, my couch, my flowers. I loved every minute of it, even the life-giving contractions! I would have liked to try a birthing pool if I had had more room at home, or a walk outside if it had not been a Michigan winter.

What would you tell an expectant mother to better prepare her for childbirth?

An expectant mother should reflect very deeply not only on how she would like to bring her child into the world, but also on how she would like to live life from that moment onwards. Birth is not the end-all; it is merely the beginning of this eternal, sacred relationship between mother and child. It is not enough to have a healthy, natural pregnancy, and then a natural birth free of unnecessary interventions. An expectant mother would be wise to read about breastfeeding, early childhood development, and child psychology. She would be wise to bring her husband with her on this educational journey, so that there will be a consensus on how their family life should be structured. Healthy parenting, the kind that goes beyond false societal norms, will be what makes a child flourish. There is a very real responsibility to overcome bad habits and to work through difficult issues before one allows them to infiltrate that sacred relationship and alter it. Indeed, birthing may come naturally to women, but child raising requires commitment to lifelong learning!

> *Birth is not the end-all; it is merely the beginning of this eternal, sacred relationship between mother and child.*

Conclusion

From Newcastle, UK to Omaha, US, women in labor are experiencing similar realities. Whether they are single mothers with no support, or married women enjoying a magnitude of encouragement from their loved ones, their childbirths are influenced by a series of factors, ranging from supportive midwives to media propaganda. Home births are rising in popularity, but remain a controversial topic. VBACs and vaginal breech births are also being requested and demanded, but are often approached by care providers with hesitation or outright refusal.

The stories shared in this book are full of emotion. There was empowerment, joy, and determination, but also sadness, fear, anxiety, and embarrassment. This was true birth. Stories told by the mothers themselves. Every single mother featured in this book reminds women to think positively about birth, and to approach it without fear. These mothers call for rights in childbirth, and for respect, dignity, and a role in decision-making. Even if oceans set them apart, these mothers are all fighting for a better birth culture. They all envision a time when expectant moms have access to the best possible medical care that can be provided. They envision a time when birth is understood as a natural phenomenon that does not require unnecessary intervention.

Our article contributors have provided us with strong, and evidence-based information and advice. These articles bring to light issues that are often sidelined or ridiculed in mainstream discussions. Topics that need to be considered in order to advance thought. Topics that deserve our attention.

Storytelling, combined with critical pieces of literature, can provide readers with something special. A resource that shows the multi-faceted dimensions of a single issue. A tool that can be used to further one's research, or to develop the courage one needs to demand a certain type of care. These two important pieces provide support and knowledge from both a professional and personal level.

From around the world, mothers have contributed their stories and articles. They have helped make this book. They have enjoyed sharing their experience with others. The discourse of childbirth is continuing because of this sharing. The discourse of childbirth must continue so that we can learn, and better understand what is needed to provide a supportive, nurturing, and respectful environment for all women giving birth.

The discourse of childbirth must continue so that we can learn, and better understand what is needed to provide a supportive, nurturing, and respectful environment for all women giving birth.

Made in the USA
Monee, IL
11 October 2020